Medical Virology

Other titles published in the Series

Anaesthetics   D. Campbell, A.A. Spence
Dermatology   J.L. Burton
Fractures and Orthopaedics   D.F. Paton
Immunology   D.M. Weir
Medical Bacteriology   J.D. Sleigh, M.C. Timbury
Medical Genetics   A.E.H. Emery
Neurology   C. Martyn
Obstetrics and Gynaecology   J. Willocks, J.P. Neilson
Ophthalmology   H.B. Chawla
Psychiatry   A. Mathews, A. Steptoe

Titles planned

Child Health
ENT
Epidemiology
General Medicine
Geriatrics
Neuroanatomy
Pharmacology
Physiology
Surgery

STUDENT NOTES

Medical Virology

Morag C. Timbury
MD PhD FRSE FRCP (Glasg.) FRCPath
Director, Central Public Health Laboratory, Public Health Laboratory Service, Colindale, London; formerly Professor of Bacteriology, University of Glasgow and Honorary Consultant Virologist, Royal Infirmary, Glasgow

NINTH EDITION

CHURCHILL LIVINGSTONE
EDINBURGH LONDON MELBOURNE AND NEW YORK 1991

CHURCHILL LIVINGSTONE
Medical Division of Longman Group UK Limited

Distributed in the United States of America by Churchill Livingstone Inc., 1560 Broadway, New York, N.Y. 10036, and by associated companies, branches and representatives throughout the world.

First edition 1967
Second edition 1969
Third edition 1971
Fourth edition 1973
Fifth edition 1974
Sixth edition 1978
Seventh edition 1983
Eighth edition 1986
Ninth edition 1991

ISBN 0-443-04148-2

British Library Cataloguing in Publication Data
CIP catalogue record for this book is available from the British Library.

Library of Congress Cataloging in Publication Data
Timbury, Morag Crichton.
    Medical virology/Morag C. Timbury. -- 9th ed.
        p. cm. -- (Student notes)
    Based on lecture notes given to the medical students at Glasgow University.
    Rev. ed. of : Notes on medical virology, 8th ed. 1986.
    Includes bibliographical references.
    Includes index.
    ISBN 0-443-04148-2
    1. Medical virology.   I. Timbury, Morag Crichton.   Notes on medical
virology.   II. Title.   III. Series.
    [DNLM: 1. Virus Diseases. 2. Viruses. WC 500 T583n]
QR201. V55T56 1991
616'. 0194--dc20
DNLM/DLC
for Library of Congress

Produced by Longman Singapore Publishers (Pte) Ltd.
Printed in Singapore

Preface

This book originated from lecture notes which were handed out to accompany my virology lectures to the medical students in Glasgow University. I wrote it in the same concise note form to try and present clearly the facts about virus diseases which students need to know for their professional examination in microbiology. Although it is meant to be reasonably comprehensive, students should refer to some of the larger books on the subject and I have listed some of my favourites on page 186.

Many colleagues have helped me with advice and discussion, notably Professor C.R. Pringle, University of Warwick, Professor A.A. Glynn, my predecessor at the Central Public Health Laboratory, and Drs P.P. Mortimer and Sylvia Gardner of the Virus Reference Laboratory here.

I should like to thank colleagues who went to considerable trouble to supply me (in previous editions) with the excellent electron micrographs and (for this edition) the colour photographs which show some of the interesting diseases that viruses cause. Thanks are due to Mr John Gibson of the Department of Medical Illustration here for his help and advice with these, and to Mr R. Callander, who prepared the drawings and diagrams. I thank, too, Mrs Kathleen Newton, who typed the manuscript for this edition.

Finally, I should like to thank Professor J.H. Subak-Sharpe for the many happy years I spent in his department, and Professor N.R. Grist in whose laboratory I first acquired my interest in viruses.

London 1991   M.C.T.

Contents

1. Viruses, general properties; disease and host response   1
2. Virus replication   15
3. Laboratory diagnosis of virus infection   29
4. Influenza   39
5. Other respiratory tract infections   47
6. Neurological diseases due to viruses   57
7. Enterovirus infections   61
8. Viral gastroenteritis   69
9. Arthropod-borne virus infections   78
10. Rabies, non-arthropod-borne haemorrhagic fevers, arenavirus infections   85
11. Herpesvirus diseases   95
12. Childhood fevers   111
13. Poxvirus diseases   123
14. Viral hepatitis   125
15. Antiviral therapy   137
16. Chronic neurological diseases due to viruses   141
17. Warts   149
18. Retroviruses   155
19. Chlamydial diseases   169
20. Rickettsial diseases   177
21. Mycoplasma   183
Recommended reading   186
Index   187

1 Viruses, general properties; disease and host response

Viruses are the smallest known infective agents. Most forms of life—animals, plants and bacteria—are susceptible to infection with appropriate viruses.

Three main properties distinguish viruses from other micro-organisms:

1. *Small size.* Viruses are smaller than other organisms, although they vary considerably in size—from 10 nm to 300 nm. In contrast, bacteria are approximately 1000 nm and erythrocytes are 7500 nm in diameter.
2. *Genome.* The genome of viruses may be either DNA or RNA; viruses contain only one kind of nucleic acid.
3. *Metabolically inert.* Viruses have no metabolic activity outside susceptible host cells; they do not possess active ribosomes or protein-synthesizing apparatus although some viruses contain enzymes within their particles; viruses cannot therefore multiply in inanimate media but only inside living cells. On entry into a susceptible cell, the virus genome or nucleic acid is transcribed into—or itself acts as—virus-specific messenger or mRNA which then directs the replication of new virus particles.

STRUCTURE OF VIRUSES

Viruses consist basically of a core of nucleic acid surrounded by a protein coat.

The protein coat protects the viral genome from inactivation by adverse environmental factors, e.g. nucleases in the blood stream. It is antigenic and often responsible for stimulating the production of protective antibodies.

The structures which make up a virus particle are known as:

Virion—the intact virus particle.

Capsid—the protein coat.

Capsomeres—the protein structural units of which the capsid is composed.

Nucleic acid

Envelope—the particles of many viruses are surrounded by a lipoprotein envelope containing viral antigens but also partly derived from the plasma or, in some cases, the nuclear membrane of the host cell.

Virus particles show three types of *symmetry*:

Cubic—in which the particles are icosahedral protein shells with the nucleic acid contained inside (Fig. 1.1).

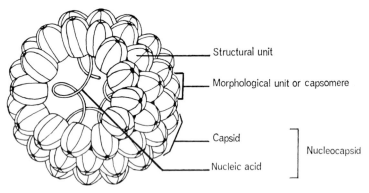

Fig. 1.1   Diagram of icosahedral virus particle with cubic symmetry.
(Reproduced, with permission, from *Virus Morphology* by C. R. Madeley.)

Helical—in which the particle contains an elongated nucleo-capsid; the capsomeres are arranged round the spiral of nucleic acid. Most helical viruses possess an outer envelope (Fig. 1.2).

Complex—in which the particle does not confirm to either cubic or helical symmetry.

CULTIVATION OF VIRUSES

Since viruses will only replicate within living cells special methods

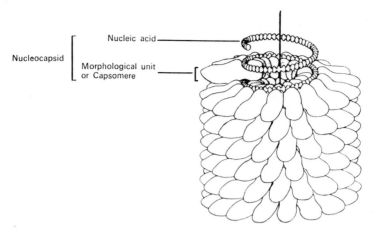

Nucleocapsid

Nucleic acid

Morphological unit
or Capsomere

Fig. 1.2   Diagram of nucleocapsid of virus particle with helical symmetry.
(Reproduced, with permission, from *Advances in Virus Research*, 1960, p. 274.)

have to be employed for culture in vitro; three main systems are used for their cultivation in the laboratory (see also Ch. 3).

1. *Tissue culture*. Cells obtained from man or animals are grown in artificial culture in glass vessels in the laboratory; the cells are living and metabolizing and so can support viral replication.

2. *Chick embryo*. Some viruses grow in the cells of the chick embryo; fertile eggs are kept in an incubator in the laboratory for this purpose. This technique has been largely superseded by tissue culture.

3. *Laboratory animals*. Before other techniques were available, viruses were isolated and studied mainly by inoculation of laboratory animals such as mice, rabbits, ferrets and monkeys; animals are still required for the isolation of a few viruses.

EFFECTS OF VIRUSES ON CELLS

Viruses may affect cells in three ways:

Cell death. The infection is lethal: it causes a cytopathic effect (CPE) which kills the cell.

Cell transformation. The cell is not killed but is changed from a normal cell to one with the properties of a malignant or cancerous cell.

Latent infection. The virus remains within the cell in a potentially active state but produces no obvious effects on the cell's functions.

Haemadsorption: some viruses have protein (haemagglutinin) in their outer coats which adheres to erythrocytes causing them to agglutinate: in tissue culture, these viruses produce haemagglutinin on the surface of infected cells to which added erythrocytes adhere.

Table 1.1   Virus classification and diseases

Family	Viruses	Diseases
DNA viruses		
Poxviruses	Variola, molluscum	Smallpox, molluscum contagiosum
Herpesviruses	Herpes simplex, varicella-zoster, cytomegalovirus, EB virus, HHV-6	Herpes, chickenpox, shingles, infectious mononucleosis
Adenoviruses	Adenoviruses	Sore throat, conjunctivitis
Hepadnavirus	Hepatitis B	Hepatitis
Papovaviruses	Papilloma, polyoma, SV_{40}	Warts, progressive multifocal leucoencephalopathy
Parvoviruses	B19	Erythema infectiosum, haemolytic crises
RNA viruses		
Orthomyxoviruses	Influenza	Influenza
Paramyxoviruses	Parainfluenza, respiratory syncytial, measles, mumps	Respiratory infection, measles, mumps
Rhabdoviruses	Rabies	Rabies
Picornaviruses	Enteroviruses, rhinoviruses, hepatitis A	Meningitis, paralysis, colds, hepatitis

Table 1.1 (Continued)

Family	Viruses	Diseases
Togaviruses	Alphaviruses, rubivirus	Encephalitis, febrile disease, rubella
Flaviruses	Flaviruses	Encephalitis, febrile disease
Bunyaviruses	Bunyaviruses, Hantaan virus	Encephalitis, febrile disease
Reoviruses	Rotavirus	Gastroenteritis
Arenaviruses	Lymphocytic choriomeningitis, Lassa virus	Meningitis, febrile disease
Retroviruses	HTLV I, II HIV-1, 2	T-cell leukaemia-lymphoma, AIDS

Note: Virus families are now known by Latin names. The more widely used anglicized names are used in this classification and throughout the text.

CLASSIFICATION

Viruses are assigned to groups mainly on the basis of the morphology of the virus particle, but also of their nucleic acid and method of RNA transcription.

A simplified scheme of classification of the main groups of medically important viruses and the diseases they cause is shown in Table 1.1. Diagrams of some representative virus particles are shown in Figure 1.3.

THE EFFECT OF PHYSICAL AND CHEMICAL AGENTS ON VIRUSES

Heat. Most are inactivated at 56°C for 30 minutes or at 100°C for a few seconds.

Cold. Stable at low temperatures, most can be stored at –40°C or, preferably, at –70°C; some viruses are partially inactivated by the process of freezing and thawing.

Drying. Variable. Some survive well, others are rapidly inactivated.

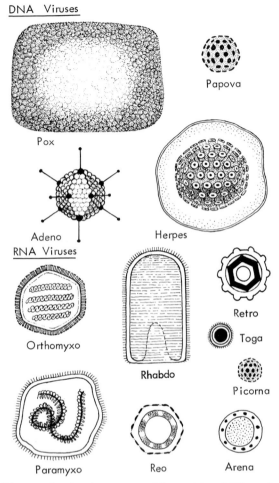

Fig. 1.3 Diagrams showing the structure of the particles of different families of virus. *Note*: These drawings are schematic and are not drawn to scale although differences in relative size are indicated.

Ultra-violet irradiation. Inactivates viruses.

Chloroform and ether. Viruses with lipid-containing envelopes are inactivated; those without envelopes are resistant.

Oxidizing and reducing agents. Viruses are inactivated by formaldehyde, chlorine, iodine and hydrogen peroxide.

β-propiolactone is used for inactivation of viruses for vaccine preparation—as is formaldehyde.

Phenols. Most viruses are relatively resistant.

Virus disinfectants. The best are hypochlorite solution (which is corrosive) and gluteraldehyde.

VIRUS DISEASES

Viruses are important and common causes of human disease, especially in children. Most viral infections are mild and the patient makes a complete recovery; many infections are silent and the virus multiplies in the body without causing symptoms of disease.

However, viral infections which are usually mild sometimes cause severe disease in an unusually susceptible patient; a few viral diseases are severe and always have a high mortality rate.

Entry

Viruses most often enter the body via the respiratory tract by *inhalation* but some viruses gain entry by *ingestion,* by *inoculation* through skin abrasions or via the bite of an *arthropod vector.*

Invasiveness

Is the main pathogenetic mechanism of viruses. Viral disease is produced by the direct spread of viruses to tissues and organs. The process of virus replication in the cells of the tissues usually— although not always— kills the infected cells. This *cytopathic effect* in vivo causes lesions and so dysfunction (and therefore symptoms and signs) in the tissue or organ concerned.

Note: In some virus infections, the immune response contributes to the pathogenesis of virus lesions. In these infections immunodeficient patients have milder or even asymptomatic infection.

HOST RESPONSE TO VIRUS INFECTION

The body defence mechanisms to virus invasions are of two types:

1. Non-specific
2. Specific

Non-specific defence mechanisms

The body has defences which are not directed at particular infectious agents, but which serve as non-immunological barriers to infection.

1. *Skin*: an effective and impermeable barrier unless breached by injury, disease, etc.
2. *Respiratory tract*: upward flow of mucus by ciliated epithelium removes virus particles to prevent invasion of the lower respiratory tract.
3. *Gastrointestinal tract*: stomach acid inactivates acid-labile viruses: bile (which lyses enveloped viruses), movement of intestinal contents and uptake of virus by lymphoid tissue aid elimination of ingested viruses.
4. *Urinary tract*: flow of urine exerts a protective flushing effect.
5. *Conjunctiva*: tears flush viruses from the eye.
6. *Phagocytosis*: an important defence mechanism in bacterial infection and probably in virus infections also: invading viruses —like bacteria—are ingested by two types of scavenger cell:
   (i) Neutrophil polymorphonuclear leucocytes
   (ii) Macrophages (or mononuclear cells of the reticuloendothelial system):
      (a) free macrophages in lung alveoli, peritoneum
      (b) fixed macrophages in lymph nodes, spleen, liver (Kupffer cells), connective tissue (histiocytes) and CNS (microglia).
   Phagocytosis is enhanced by antibody (which is of course, a specific immune mechanism) and complement: this effect is known as *opsonisation*.
   'Activated' macrophages—due to lymphokines from T_d lymphocytes (a specific immune mechanism)—have increased phagocytic activity and are attracted by chemotaxis to the site of infection
7. *Interferons*: a mechanism in part stimulated by the immune response by which the body overcomes acute virus infection.

Specific immunological defence mechanisms

Immunological responses are of two types:

	Main effect
1. Humoral	Elimination of infectious virus
2. Cellular	Elimination of virus-infected cells

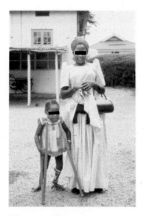

Plate 1 Poliomyelitis. Child with residual paralysis and wasting in affected leg. (Photograph by Dr Eric Walker.)

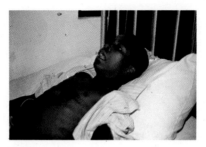

Plate 2 Rabies. Patient in hydrophobic spasm. (Photograph by Dr D. A. Warrell.)

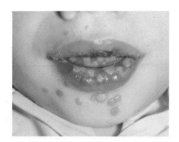

Plate 3 Primary herpes simplex infection. Stomatitis with satellite vesicles over the chin. (Reproduced, with permission, from *Diseases of Infection* by N.R. Grist, D.O. Ho-Yen, E. Walker and G.R. Williams, 1988. Oxford University Press.)

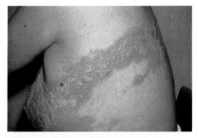

Plate 4 Zoster. Thoracic rash with characteristic distribution of lesions, 'a belt of roses from hell'. (Photograph by Dr Alan Lyell.)

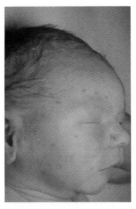

Plate 5 Congenital rubella. Purpuric rash in newborn infant with congenitally-acquired rubella, who was subsequently found to have congenital heart disease and cataract as well. (Reproduced with permission from Topley and Wilson's *Principles of Bacteriology, Virology and Immunity*, Vol 4, 7th edition, 1984. Edward Arnold, London.)

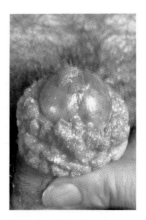

Plate 6 Genital warts. Large penile warts caused by papillomavirus. (Photograph by The Photography and Illustration Centre, The Middlesex Hospital.)

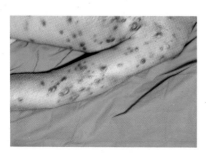

Plate 7 AIDS. The characteristic purplish skin tumours of Kaposi's sarcoma. (Photograph by The Photography and Illustration Centre, The Middlesex Hospital.)

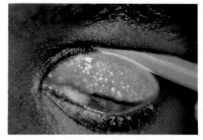

Plate 8 Trachoma. Showing severe follicular hyperplasia and papillary hyperplasia in the conjunctiva. (Photograph by the late Mr Josef Sowa. Reproduced with permission of the Controller of Her Majesty's Stationery Office, from MRC Special Research Series Report No. 308.)

Humoral

Like other infectious agents, viruses provoke production of anti-bodies in the blood. Antibodies are:

(i) *Immunoglobulins*: proteins which react specifically with antigens—which are also usually proteins—in virus particles

(ii) *Produced by plasma cells*: formed when B-lymphocytes are activated by encounter with antigen. B-lymphocytes have immunoglobulin on their surface which acts as receptor for virus antigen. T-helper cells contribute to the differentiation of B cells to plasma cells.

(iii) *Structure*: is Y-shaped. The stem is the Fc fragment which activates complement and binds to receptors on infected host cells: the two arms are the Fab fragments and contain the antibody-combining sites.

There are three main immunoglobulins responsible for humoral immunity in virus infections:

(i) *IgM*: the earliest antibody produced: formed about a week after infection, it persists for about 4–6 weeks: a pentamer of five IgG molecules

(ii) *IgG*: formed later than IgM but persists for months and often years: responsible for the immunity to reinfection

(iii) *IgA*: a dimeric molecule: found in body secretions as well as blood, i.e. saliva, respiratory secretions, tears and intestinal contents: the IgA in secretions acquires a carbohydrate 'transport piece' in extracellular fluids but this is absent in serum IgA: IgA is the main antibody responsible for immunity to respiratory viruses and for the gut immunity seen after enteric virus infection

Antiviral effects:

1. **Neutralization:** antiviral antibodies neutralize virus infectivity: neutralizing antibody is the principal mechanism for the immunity—often lifelong—which follows virus infection and prevents re-infection.
   Neutralization is the principal mechanism for the elimination of infectious virus.
   Complement: enhances the neutralizing effect of antibody
2. **Antibody-dependent cell-mediated cytotoxicity** (see below).

Cellular

Cellular immunity is increasingly recognized as the most important body defence against viruses. For example, children with
congenital deficiency of cellular immunity are abnormally susceptible to virus infection and often (although not always) develop
unusually severe disease: those with humoral immune deficiency,
on the other hand, respond to virus infections like normal
children. **Cellular immunity is the mechanism for elimination of virus-infected cells.**

Mediated by T or thymus-dependent lymphocytes.

Four types of lymphocyte are involved:
cytotoxic T cells (T_c cells)
helper T cells (T_h cells)
suppressor T cells (T_s cells)
delayed hypersensitivity T cells (T_d cells).

Cell-mediated immune response to virus. Principally
directed against virus-infected cells, the response is extremely
complex and involves other elements, cells and lymphokines, in
addition to lymphocytes. Below is a simplified version:

Virus is recognized as antigen by T_h cells when presented by
a macrophage acting as an antigen-presenting cell: recognition is
dependent on the Class II MHC, i.e. major histocompatibility
(DR) antigens of the macrophage being compatible with those on
the T_h cells.

Interleukin-1 (IL-1) is released from antigen-presenting cells:
it induces receptors for a second lymphokine—IL-2—on a subset
of T cells and also the production of IL-2 itself, which then
stimulates the receptor-bearing cells to proliferate.

T_h or helper lymphocytes generally stimulate the cytotoxic
cellular response and cause activation of B cells (the antibody-
producing cells): these effects are produced by secretion of the
lymphokine IL-2.

T_s or suppressor lymphocytes, on the other hand, control
and regulate the cytotoxic cellular response by suppression of T_h
cells. They are probably also responsible for immune *tolerance* to
foreign antigens.

T_c or cytotoxic lymphocytes are the main effector cells
which kill virus-infected target cells: Class I MHC antigen com-

patibility is required for this, i.e. the cells are Class I MHC restricted: T_c cells react directly with virus antigens expressed on the surface of the infected cell.

T_d or delayed type hypersensitivity cells: release macrophage activation factor.

Lysis of virus-infected cells is mediated by several mechanisms:

1. Antibody-independent or direct killing by:
   (i) T_c cells
   (ii) Natural killer (NK) cells—these are also lymphocytes (but with a granular appearance) and are present in the non-immune host.
2. Antibody-dependent—known as antibody dependent cellular cytolysis or ADCC: mediated via Fc binding between the Fc portion of antiviral IgG bound to virus on cell surfaces and Fc receptors on:
   (i) Killer (K) cells—lymphocytes present in non-immune as as well as immune hosts
   (ii) Polymorphonuclear leucocytes
   (iii) Activated macrophages

This complex of immunological reactions is the major body defence which localizes and eliminates the acute virus infection with the response directed towards the destruction of virus-infected cells. Activated macrophages (see above) also play a part in this process. Clearly antibody has a role in the cellular response, but also aids the elimination of virus directly through its specific and effective neutralizing activity.

INTERFERONS

There are three main classes of interferons:

Interferon	Cell of origin	Number of subtypes
α	Leucocyte	12
β	Fibroblast	1
γ	Lymphocyte	1

Originally regarded as primarily a defence mechanism against viruses, interferons are now thought to resemble a family of hormones with wide and various modulatory effects, including an anti-proliferative activity on cells and the immune system, as well as on virus replication.

Interferons have the following properties:

1. *Host specific*: so that only human interferon is fully active in human cells
2. *Wide antiviral spectrum*: most viruses are inhibited
3. *Induction*
   (i) α and β interferons are induced by viruses and synthetic double-stranded RNA (which may mimic an intermediate product in virus replication)
   (ii) γ interferon is induced by antigenic stimulation of lymphocytes: it can be regarded as a lymphokine.
4. *Action*
   (i) site—interferons bind to receptors on the cell surface
   (ii) induction of enzymes:
   2–5 A synthetase
   RNAase L (an endoribonuclease)
   Protein kinase (inactivates the peptide chain initiation factor (eIF-2))
   (iii) inhibition of virus replication: cells treated with interferon are refractory to virus infection: both virus transcription and protein synthesis are prevented

Note: interferon acts as a lymphokine to activate macrophages and to amplify the action of natural killer cells.

Role of interferons

Interferons have powerful antiviral activity and are part of the immediate body response to invasion by viruses. They can be demonstrated in blood and tissues during the acute phase of virus infections. It seems likely that antiviral defence is the main function of α and β interferons, but interferons also inhibit cell proliferation and so have clearly a wider role in body regulatory mechanisms. γ interferon has had clinical trials as an anti-cancer agent.

Antiviral chemotherapy

Interferon has been genetically engineered and can now be obtained in large quantities and in pure form. Although long thought to be potentially an ideal chemotherapeutic agent against viruses, its potential has not been realised in practice. Side effects (similar to those of pyrogen) have proved troublesome and despite undoubted clinical response with some viruses, its applications are fairly restricted and fall far short of initial hopes and expectations.

2 Virus replication

Viruses have no metabolic activity of their own: they replicate by taking over the biochemical machinery of the host cell and redirecting it to the manufacture of virus components. This take-over is achieved by *virus mRNA*.

VIRUS GROWTH CYCLE

Takes place in seven stages:

1. **Adsorption**
    (i) to specific receptors on the cell plasma membrane
    (ii) best at 37°C but also—although slowly—at 4°C
    (iii) enhanced by Mg^{++} or Ca^{++}.
2. **Entry**
    (i) complex: probably by invagination of cell membrane round virus particle to enclose it in a pinocytotic vacuole
    (ii) with syncytia-producing viruses by fusion of virus envelope with cell membrane.
3. **Uncoating**
    (i) releases—or renders accessible—the virus nucleic acid or genome
    (ii) cell enzymes (from lysosomes) strip off the virus protein coat.
4. **Transcription**
    (i) the production of virus mRNA or replicative intermediates from the viral genome
    (ii) carried out either by host cell or virus-specified enzyme
    (iii) subject to complex control mechanisms:
        a. patterns of transcription often differ before (early) and after (late) virus nucleic acid replication
        b. many virus genomes contain *promoters* and *enhancers* that stimulate transcription

    c. primary transcripts are often spliced to remove intron sequences between expressed exons

    d. transcription sometimes overlaps with different starting and/or termination points within one gene to produce different proteins from the same nucleic acid sequence.

Virus mRNA generally, but not invariably:

(i) contains leader sequences

(ii) capped at the 5′ end

(iii) polyadenylated at the 3′ terminus

5. **Synthesis of virus components**

Virus protein synthesis: virus mRNA is translated on cell ribosomes into two types of virus protein:

    a. structural—the proteins which make up the virus particle

    b. non-structural—not found in the particle, mainly enzymes for virus genome replication.

Virus nucleic acid synthesis:

(i) new virus genomes are synthesized

(ii) templates are either the parental genome or, with single-stranded nucleic acid genomes, newly formed complementary strands

(iii) most often by a virus-coded polymerase or replicase: with some DNA viruses a cell enzyme carries this out.

6. **Assembly**

(i) new virus genomes and proteins are assembled to form new virus particles

(ii) may take place in cell nucleus, cytoplasm or (with most enveloped viruses) at the plasma membrane which invests the new particle to form the virus envelope.

7. **Release**

(i) either by sudden rupture or by gradual extrusion (budding) of enveloped viruses through the cell membranes.

VIRUS GENOMES

Nucleic acid

(i) may be DNA or RNA

(ii) single- or double-stranded

(iii) intact or fragmented, linear or circular

(iv) some viruses (adeno and polio) have a small protein covalently bonded to the 5′ terminus.

Table 2.1 Some properties of viruses and their genomes

Virus family	Example	Type[a]	Nucleic Acid		Transcriptase contained in virus particles
			Molecular weight ($\times 10^6$)	Infectivity	
Pox	Vaccinia	DS DNA	160	0	+
Herpes	Herpes simplex	DS DNA	100	+	0
Adeno	Adenovirus	DS DNA	23	+	0
Papova	Polyoma	DS DNA	3	+	0
Hepadnavirus	Hepatitis B	DS DNA	2.3	0	+[e]
Parvo	B 19	SS DNA	1.7	+	0
Picorna	Poliovirus	SS RNA	2.6	+	0
Calici	Feline calicivirus	SS RNA	2.7	+	0
Toga	Sindbis	SS RNA	4	+	0
Corona	Coronavirus	SS RNA	5.8	+	0
Orthomyxo	Influenza A	SS RNA[c]	5.7	0	+
Paramyxo	Parainfluenza	SS RNA	7	0	+
Arena	Lassa fever	SS RNA[c]	3.2	0	+
Bunya	Crimean haemorrhagic fever	SS RNA[c]	6.4	0	+
Rhabdo	Rabies	SS RNA	4	0	+
Retro	HIV-1	SS RNA[d]	3	0[e]	+[b]
Reovirus	Rotavirus	DS RNA[c]	11	0	+

[a] DS = double-stranded; SS = single-stranded
[b] reverse transcriptase
[c] fragmented (reovirus 11 unique sub-units, orthomyxo 8, bunya 3, arena 2)
[d] two identical sub-units in the virion
[e] virion contains DNA polymerase and reverse transcriptase

Large viruses

(i) have high molecular weight nucleic acid
(ii) code for many proteins
(iii) code for many of the enzymes involved in replication.

Small viruses

(i) have low molecular weight nucleic acid
(ii) therefore limited coding capacity
(iii) must use some of the cell enzymes for replication.

Infectivity

(i) with many viruses the purified nucleic acid genome is infectious when applied to cells—i.e. without the capsid, nucleic acid on its own can infect a cell to initiate a complete infectious cycle of virus replication

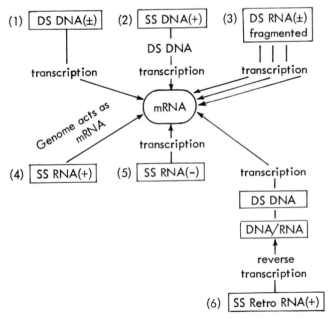

Fig. 2.1 Diagram to show methods of transcription of the six different groups in the Baltimore classification of virus genomes.

(ii) virus genomes of which the virions contain a transcriptase are non-infectious: this is because the process of nucleic acid extraction removes the virion transcriptase and mRNA cannot then be produced.

The properties of the main virus groups and their genomes are shown in Table 2.1.

Baltimore classification

This classifies viruses into six groups on the basis of their nucleic acid and mRNA production (Fig. 2.1).

BIOCHEMISTRY OF VIRUS REPLICATION

An extremely complex subject: a few examples only will be outlined here to highlight the main differences in the growth cycles of some representative group of viruses.

Double-stranded DNA viruses

Examples: vaccinia, herpes simplex, adeno, polyoma viruses. The principal steps in their growth cycle are detailed below and shown diagrammatically in Figure 2.2.

Transcription: two main types of mRNA are produced:

1. *Early* mRNA—before virus DNA synthesis—codes mainly for enzymes required for DNA synthesis
2. *Late* mRNA—after virus DNA synthesis—codes mainly for structural proteins.

Virus DNA synthesis:

Enzymes: many are involved but

1. the main DNA replicative enzyme is DNA-dependent DNA polymerase
2. larger viruses code for their own enzyme (vaccinia, herpes simplex)
3. smaller viruses use the host cell DNA polymerase (adenovirus, polyoma).

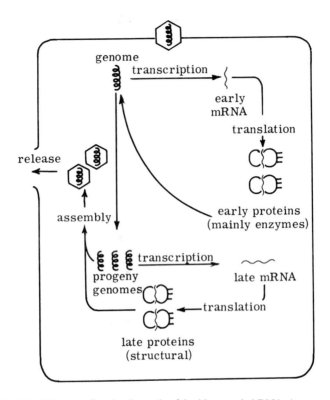

Fig. 2.2   Diagram of replicative cycle of double-stranded DNA virus.

Template: new progeny virus DNA is synthesized off the DNA genome of the input parental virus.

Site: nucleus (except pox viruses)

New progeny DNA: acts as templates for:

1. transcription of late virus mRNA
2. synthesis of more genomes for new virus particles.

Virus protein synthesis: is a two-stage process:

1. production of early proteins required for virus DNA synthesis (e.g. DNA-dependent DNA polymerase, thymidine kinase, other enzymes)
2. production of late proteins

(i) produced after virus DNA synthesis
(ii) mostly the capsid proteins for new particles.

Site: virus proteins are synthesized on the ribosomes in the cell cytoplasm and then transported to sites of assembly.

Assembly: of new DNA genomes and proteins into new infectious particles within the cell takes place in:

1. *Nucleus*—herpes simplex, adeno, polyoma viruses:
   Note: herpes particles acquire an envelope by budding through the cell nuclear membrane which has been modified by the incorporation within it of virus glycoproteins.
2. *Cytoplasm*—vaccinia replicates entirely in the cytoplasm in 'factories' which are based on clusters of ribosomes.

Other DNA viruses

Hepatitis B virus has an unusual and complex replication cycle. The infectious particle contains an incompletely double-stranded DNA molecule and a DNA polymerase which can fill in the gap to produce a complete double-stranded molecule. The genes for the surface and core proteins overlap (and presumably so too does the gene for the DNA polymerase). Replication of the genome is unique in that it appears to involve a negative strand RNA template generated by reverse transcription to produce an RNA/DNA intermediate which is subsequently converted to double-stranded DNA.

Parvoviruses—for example, B19 virus—have a tiny single-stranded DNA genome. Some are *autonomous* in replication (eg. human parvovirus), others are *defective* and require a helper virus for replication (eg. adeno-associated virus which is dependent on a helper adenovirus). Autonomous parvoviruses generally package within their virions only minus or negative strand DNA (i.e. strands from which virus mRNA is transcribed): defective viruses package both plus and minus strand DNA but separately within different particles. Both autonomous and defective viruses have terminally redundant DNA but in the former the repeated regions are different whereas with the defective viruses they have identical sequences. The parvovirus genome codes for three structural proteins from overlapping sequences.

RNA viruses

Because their genetic material is RNA, these viruses use biochemical mechanisms for their replication which are different from those of other forms of living organisms. RNA virus genomes have different methods of transcription:

1. *Single-strand positive sense RNA*: the virus genome is the virus mRNA
2. *Single-strand negative sense RNA*: virus mRNA is transcribed from the parental genome
3. *Double-stranded fragmented RNA*: individual virus mRNAs are transcribed separately off the parental RNA segments using a transcriptase associated with each segment
4. *Retrovirus*: the virus genome alternates between RNA and DNA: parental single-stranded RNA is transcribed into double-stranded DNA and integrated into the host genome as a 'provirus' from which virus RNA is later transcribed. But note, retrovirus genomes are inverted dimers of two complete genomes.

Below are selected examples of the replication cycle of some RNA viruses.

Single-stranded positive sense RNA viruses

Example: poliovirus.

With these viruses, there is no transcription stage because the single-stranded positive sense RNA acts itself as virus mRNA. The replication cycle is shown diagrammatically in Figure 2.3.

Translation

The virus genome is translated into one very large polypeptide which is almost immediately cleaved into smaller proteins as follows:

1. structural viral capsid proteins
2. the RNA-dependent RNA polymerase required for replication of virus RNA (no similar enzyme exists in cells)
3. a protease for cleaving the precursor polypeptide
4. a genome-linked terminal protein.

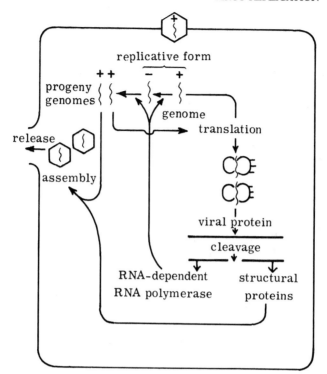

Fig. 2.3 Diagram of replicative cycle of single-stranded positive sense RNA virus.

Virus RNA synthesis

New genome production takes place on a double-stranded 'replicative form' made by the synthesis of a negative sense RNA strand complementary to the input positive sense parental RNA.

New progeny positive sense RNA strands are synthesized off the template of the negative RNA strand in the replicative form.

RNA-dependent RNA polymerase synthesizes both the replicative form and also new positive sense RNA strand genomes.

Progeny positive sense RNA functions as:

1. templates for the production of more replicative forms (and so for more genome RNA synthesis)

2. genomes for new virus particles
3. virus mRNA.

Assembly

New progeny virus particles are assembled from the cleavage products of the primary translation product and from progeny virus RNA in the cytoplasm on clusters of ribosomes: poliovirus replicates entirely in the cytoplasm.

Release

By sudden rupture of the cell.

Single-stranded negative sense RNA viruses

Example: parainfluenza virus.
   The replicative cycle is shown diagrammatically in Figure 2.4.

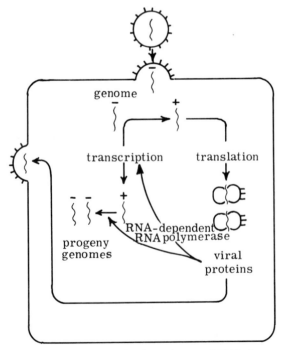

Fig. 2.4   Diagram of replicative cycle of negative strand RNA virus.

Transcription

Virus mRNA is synthesized off the parental (negative sense strand) genome RNA using a transcriptase (RNA-dependent RNA polymerase) contained in the virus particle.

Separate virus mRNAs are produced for each of the different virus proteins.

Virus RNA synthesis

Virus progeny genomes are produced—also by the transcriptase—using RNA positive sense strands complementary to the parental genome as templates.

Virus protein synthesis

Virus proteins include:

1. transcriptase
2. envelope proteins (two are glycosylated and have haemag-glutinin/neuraminidase and fusion/haemolysis activities respectively)
3. nucleocapsid proteins.

Assembly

New virus nucleocapsids are assembled at the cell membrane and become enveloped by budding through the plasma membrane.

Note: influenza virus has a fragmented genome each fragment of which codes for a different virus protein.

Double-stranded RNA viruses

Example: reoviruses.

All double-stranded RNA viruses have *fragmented genomes*. Each fragment codes for a different protein and each is associated with a molecule of transcriptase (RNA-dependent RNA polymerase). The replicative cycle starts with transcription of mRNA from each double-stranded RNA fragment—the mRNAs produced then being translated into the different virus proteins. These mRNA molecules later become enclosed within nucleocapsids together with a transcriptase which directs the synthesis of a complementary RNA strand to produce the double-stranded fragments which make up the genome.

Retrovirus

Example: HIV-1

Retroviruses are tumour viruses which can replicate in cells without killing them and may also *transform* normal cells into malignant or cancer cells. Their replication involves the production of virus DNA which integrates into the cell chromosome.

The retrovirus genome: is single-stranded dimeric RNA with three principal genes and with long terminal repeat regions which enable integration—in the DNA provirus form—into the host cell chromosome. The long terminal repeats contain promoter sequences. The three principal genes are:

1. *gag*—core proteins
2. *pol*—polymerase—i.e. reverse transcriptase (contained in the virion)
3. *env*—envelope proteins.

The replicative cycle is shown diagrammatically in Figure 2.5.

First stage:
1. *transcription* (by the reverse transcriptase contained in the virion) to produce a DNA/RNA genome heteroduplex.
2. *conversion* of the DNA/RNA heteroduplex into double-stranded DNA.
3. *integration* of the double-stranded virus DNA into the cellular chromosome where it is known as *provirus*.

Second stage:
1. provirus DNA is transcribed (by cell enzyme)
2. the RNA transcripts produced have two functions—
   (i) *mRNA* for translation into virus proteins
   (ii) new virus genomes.

Virus protein synthesis: virus proteins are produced on cell ribosomes by translation of mRNA transcribed off the provirus DNA.

1. reverse transcriptase
2. core proteins
3. envelope proteins.

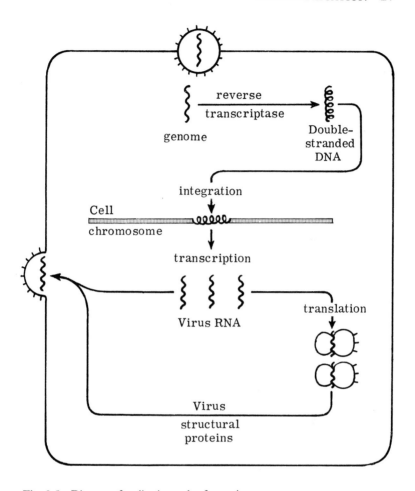

Fig. 2.5 Diagram of replicative cycle of retrovirus.

Assembly: virus nucleocapsids are assembled from the progeny virus RNA genomes and proteins at the cell surface and acquire their outer envelope by budding through the cell plasma membrane.

3 Laboratory diagnosis of virus infection

Virus diseases are diagnosed by:

1. **Serology**, i.e. demonstration of virus antibody
2. **Isolation** of virus
3. **Direct demonstration** of virus or antigen in material from the patient.

SEROLOGY

Serological diagnosis depends on the detection of virus antibody and is by far the most widely used way to diagnose virus infection.

Detection of virus antibody

Virus antibodies are common in healthy populations and can remain at a high level for many years after infection. A diagnosis of recent infection depends on the following criteria:

1. *Detection of IgM*: the earliest antibody to appear and therefore only present if there has been recent infection. Increasingly used as a method of diagnosis. Detect using anti-human IgM and test serum against virus antigen by enzyme-linked immunoabsorbent assay (ELISA) or immunofluorescence (see below).

2. *Rising titre*: i.e. increase in the level of antibody (at least four-fold) over the course of infection from the acute phase into convalescence.

Note: titre is the highest dilution of an antiserum at which activity is demonstrated: usually expressed as the reciprocal of the antiserum dilution, i.e. 64 rather than 1/64.

3. *High stationary titre*: unreliable: but if the titre of antibody is *considerably* higher than that found in the general population, recent infection with the virus can be assumed.

Tests used in serology

The old but well-tried and reliable technique of complement fixation test is now being replaced by more sensitive assays—especially those which detect virus-specific IgM. But, note, the complement fixation test is still an indispensable technique in virus laboratories.

Below are some of the most widely used tests:

1. **Enzyme-linked immunoabsorbent assay (ELISA)**: Now widely used and often available as commercially produced kits. It is more economical in terms of staff time than immuno-flourescence and can be automated. Note, however, that ELISA tests are not really quantitative, unless the serum under test is diluted to determine the end point dilution at which a positive reaction is observed—a tedious and often expensive process.

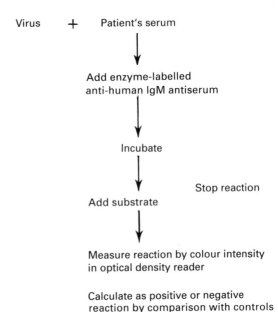

Fig. 3.1   Diagram for ELISA test for virus IgM antibody.

Anti-human IgM (or anti-IgG) antibody is used to detect specific IgM (or IgG) in the serum under test (Fig. 3.1). Labelled anti-human antibody is used to detect the virus antibody: the label is an enzyme which reacts with a suitable substrate to produce a visible colour change. The enzyme substrates most often used are:

(i) Horseradish peroxidase and hydrogen peroxide: ortho-phenyldiamine

(ii) Alkaline phosphatase: paranitrophenyl phosphate.

2. **Radioimmunoassay (RIA)**: Generally the most sensitive technique. Similar in principle to ELISA but the detecting anti-human antibody is tagged with an isotope—most often I^{125}.

Radioisotopes can only be handled in specially designed and equipped laboratories. As a result RIA is less widely used than other serological tests.

Antibody capture tests: Both ELISA and RIA tests can be made more sensitive and more specific by 'capturing' patient's IgM, reacting it with virus and then by adding labelled monoclonal antiviral antibody. This is illustrated in Figure 3.2.

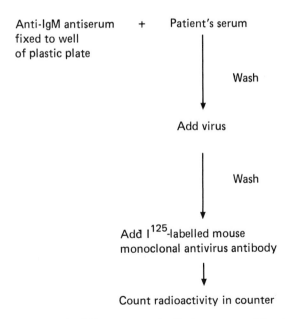

Fig. 3.2   Diagram of radioimmunoassay (antibody capture test) for virus IgM antibody.

3. **Complement fixation test**: Virus antibody is detected by the fixation of added complement when the antibody combines with virus antigen. The fixation is rendered visible by later addition of sheep erythrocytes sensitized by addition of anti-erythrocyte antibody (Fig. 3.3). If virus antibody is present complement is fixed and the sheep red cells do not haemolyse: if no virus antibody is present the complement lyses the sensitized erythrocytes.

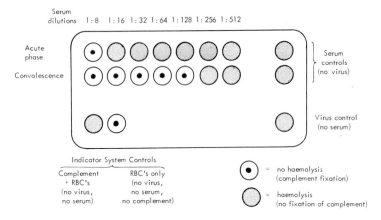

Fig. 3.3   Diagram for complement fixation test for viral antibody. Virus antigen is mixed overnight at 4°C with dilutions of the patient's serum and complement before addition of sensitized sheep erythrocytes. Titre of complement-fixing antibody has risen from 8 in the acute phase to 128 in convalescence—a greater than 4-fold rise in titre indicating recent infection.

4. **Immunofluorescence**: Virus-specific antibody is detected usually by the indirect or sandwich technique. In this, dilutions of patient's serum are added to spots of virus-infected cells on microscope slides. After washing, virus antibody is detected on the cells by application of fluorescein-labelled anti-human IgG or IgM. Fluorescence is detected by examination in a microscope under ultraviolet light and indicates the presence of virus antibody and—according to the highest dilution of the patient's serum at which this is observed—the titre of antibody. Sometimes virus antibody is detected by addition of complement to the reaction and then detecting its fixation by fluorescein-labelled anti-complement antibody.

5. **Haemagglutination-inhibition test**: Many viruses haemagglutinate erythrocytes but virus antibody blocks this. Antibody can be detected in a patient's serum by inhibition of virus haemagglutination (Fig. 3.4).

6. **Radial immune haemolysis**: A useful qualitative test for antibody detection—but not titration—with haemagglutinating viruses. Widely used as a screen test for immunity to rubella. Virus and erythrocytes are mixed in an agar gel in a plate with added complement. Patient's sera are added to wells cut in the agar: if antibody is present, zones of haemolysis appear round the wells on incubation.

7. **Neutralization**: Antibody prevents virus infection of cells. Antibody can be detected by neutralization of virus cytopathic effect (CPE) in tissue culture. Time-consuming and labour-intensive so not widely used.

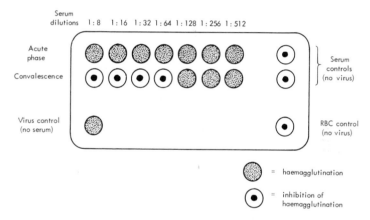

Fig. 3.4   Diagram of haemagglutination-inhibition test for viral antibody. The haemagglutinating virus is mixed with dilutions of the patient's serum for one hour before addition to erythrocytes. Titre of haemagglutination-inhibiting antibody has risen from less than 8 in the acute phase to 64 in convalescence—a greater than 4-fold rise in titre indicating recent infection.

VIRUS ISOLATION

Virus isolation requires the use of living cells since viruses cannot grow on inanimate media. There are three main systems:

1. Tissue culture

2. Chick embryo
3. Laboratory animals } now rarely used.

1. Tissue culture

Tissue culture is really cell culture in vitro and consists of a single layer (monolayer) of actively metabolizing cells adherent to a glass or plastic surface in a test tube, petri plate or on one side of a bottle.

The main types of tissue culture are:

1. *Primary cultures*: are laborious to prepare and short-lived but generally susceptible to a wide range of viruses. There is little cell division and although one subculture can be done, the cells die in about two to three weeks, e.g. monkey kidney.

2. *Semi-continuous cell strains*: are established from human embryo lung: easy to maintain and can be subcultured for about 30 to 40 passages before the cells die off. Susceptible to a wide range of viruses.

3. *Continuous cell lines*: can be subcultured indefinitely and are therefore easy to maintain. Generally susceptible to fewer viruses than the other types of cell culture. HeLa (derived from human cervical cancer) is the most widely known.

Medium: cells are grown in chemically defined media which are balanced and buffered salt solutions with added amino acids and vitamins. Serum is always required—generally 10% (by volume) of calf serum (or sometimes fetal calf serum for delicate cells). Penicillin and streptomycin are included to prevent bacterial contamination.

Atmosphere: because the main buffer in the medium is bicarbonate, cells produce carbon dioxide: if this is lost to the air, e.g. in open petri plates, the pH of the medium becomes alkaline and kills the cells. Tissue cultures are therefore grown in stoppered test tubes or screw-capped bottles or, if in petri plates, in an incubator with the atmosphere enriched with 5 to 10% carbon dioxide.

Temperature: the optimal temperature is 37°C.

Specimens

Material from lesions or sites of infection can be conveniently collected on a wooden-shafted swab. The tip of the swab is broken off into a bottle of transport medium. Virus laboratories supply these on request.

Delivery: should be prompt as many viruses die off rapidly at room temperature. If delay is unavoidable, keep the specimen at 4°C (e.g. in a domestic refrigerator).

Inoculation: a small volume of virus in transport medium, vesicle or other fluid or an extract in buffer solution of tissue or excretion, is added to the medium of a tube of tissue culture.

Virus growth is recognized by:

1. *CPE* (cytopathic effect): the virus kills the cells which round up and fall off the glass (Fig. 3.5). Some viruses cause cell fusion and their growth is recognized by the appearance of syncytia.

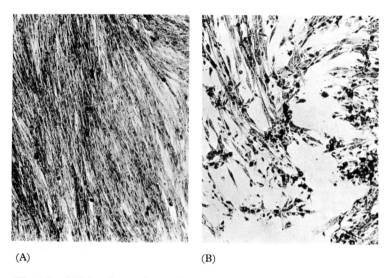

(A)   (B)

Fig. 3.5   CPE in a tissue culture of fibroblastic cells. (A) Uninoculated control. (B) Culture showing viral CPE.

2. *Haemadsorption*: added erythrocytes adhere to the surface of infected cells with haemagglutinating virus (Fig 3.6): sometimes virus can be detected by haemagglutination in the medium (Fig. 3.7).

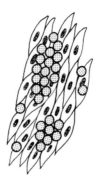

Fig. 3.6   Diagram of haemadsorption: clumps of erythrocytes are adhering to infected cells in the tissue culture.

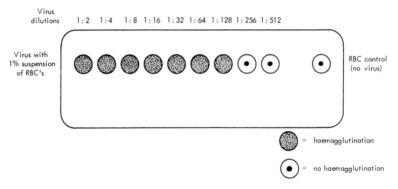

Fig. 3.7   Diagram of haemagglutination test for virus. Titre of virus haemagglutinin is 128.

3. *Immunofluorescence*: infected cells are detected by fluorescence.

Identification: the virus isolated is identified serologically by neutralization of the CPE (or of haemagglutination) with standard antiviral serum: immunofluorescence (with standard or monoclonal viral antibody) or electron microscopy is also used.

2. Chick embryo

Rarely used now for virus diagnosis. Useful for preparation of bulk virus, e.g. for antigen or vaccine production.

3. Laboratory animals

Some viruses can only be isolated by inoculation of laboratory animals, usually mice. After inoculation the animals are observed for signs of disease or death. The viruses are identified by testing for neutralization of their pathogenicity for animals by standard antiviral sera.

DIRECT DEMONSTRATION OF VIRUS

This is now becoming a widely used—and fast—method of virus diagnosis. Virus or virus antigen is detected in lesions, fluids, tissues or excretions from the patient and a result can be obtained within an hour or two of receipt of the specimen. The main techniques are:

1. *Serological*: preferably with monoclonal antiviral antibody. The most popular method is immunofluorescence; ELISA is now also being used for this: especially useful for rapid diagnosis of respiratory virus infection.

2. *Electron microscopy*: virus particles are detected and can be provisionally identified (but not serologically typed) on the basis of their morphology. Widely used—indeed indispensable—for detection of the faecal viruses that cause gastroenteritis.

3. *Probes*: Radioactive virus DNA can be used to detect virus genome or mRNA in tissues and fluids by molecular hybridization: still largely an experimental technique but of great potential value, particularly for investigation of pathology of virus disease. The polymerase chain reaction (PCR) technique provides a powerful tool for amplification of virus nucleic acid in tissues, cells, body fluids, etc.

Inclusion bodies: are virus-induced masses seen in the nucleus or cytoplasm of infected cells. With a few exceptions they are too non-specific to be useful in diagnosis.

4 Influenza

Influenza is one of the great epidemic diseases. From time to time, influenza becomes pandemic and sweeps throughout the world. The most severe pandemic recorded was in the winter of 1918 to 1919, when more than 20 million people perished. World-wide pandemics of influenza are due to the emergence of antigenically new strains of influenza virus to which there is no pre-existing immunity.

Clinical features

Route of infection: inhalation of respiratory secretions from an infected person.

Incubation period: from 1 to 4 days.

Signs and symptoms: fever, malaise, headaches, generalized aches, sometimes with nasal discharge and sneezing; a non-productive hacking cough is common and there may be sore throat and hoarseness.

Duration: symptoms usually last for about 4 days but tiredness and weakness often persists for longer.

Primary site of virus multiplication: superficial epithelium of the upper but especially the lower respiratory tract. Influenza causes damage to the cilia and desquamation of the epithelium.

Complications

In a small proportion of cases the acute infection progresses to pneumonia: two kinds of pneumonia may follow influenza:

1. *Primary influenzal pneumonia*, in which the condition of a patient with typical influenza suddenly deteriorates with the onset

of severe respiratory distress and symptoms of hypoxia, dyspnoea and cyanosis; circulatory collapse follows and the patient almost always dies. Post mortem, there is congestion of the lungs with desquamation of ciliated epithelium and hyperaemia of tracheal and bronchial mucosa; no significant bacteria are present.

2. *Secondary bacterial pneumonia*, usually develops later in the course of influenza and is due to secondary invasion of the lungs by bacteria such as *Staphylococcus aureus*, *Haemophilus influenzae* or pneumococci. The signs and symptoms are those of severe bacterial pneumonia; although there is a high mortality rate, the disease is less lethal than primary influenzal pneumonia. Post mortem there is heavy invasion of the lungs by bacteria.

Reye's syndrome

This is a rare complication sometimes seen in children after influenza (and other virus infections also); there is cerebral oedema and fatty degeneration of the viscera—especially the liver—which results in raised transaminase levels in the blood; there is a high mortality rate. *Aspirin* may predispose to the syndrome and children should therefore not be treated with this drug.

Types of virus

There are three influenza viruses, A, B and C, which can be differentiated by complement fixation test:

A—the principal cause of epidemic influenza
B—usually associated with a milder disease but also causes winter epidemics
C—of doubtful pathogenicity for man.

Influenza A viruses are also found in animals—notably birds, pigs and horses.

Epidemiology

Seasonal distribution: infection is most prevalent during the winter (but the epidemic of 'Asian' influenza started in Britain in the summer of 1957).

Spread: is more rapid than with any other infectious disease: in addition to other important properties, influenza virus possesses an inherent capacity for rapid spread.

Epidemics: pandemics of influenza A break out every few years and the epidemic strain spreads world-wide. The most severe epidemic with a high mortality rate was in 1918–19 and was due to a virus related to swine influenza A virus; unlike most influenza outbreaks this caused a high mortality amongst young adults: usually influenza is most severe in the elderly or in patients with chronic respiratory or cardiac disease.

Epidemic spread: is associated with antigenic change in the haemagglutinin on the virus surface—which is the main antigen involved in virus neutralization (see below).

Virology

1. Orthomyxoviruses ('myxo' = affinity for mucin)
2. RNA viruses—the RNA is in eight separate single-stranded, negative sense fragments each of which is a gene and codes for a different protein, e.g. the haemagglutinin, the neuraminidase, etc.

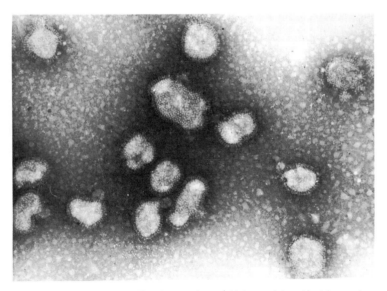

Fig. 4.1 Influenza virus. The virus nucleocapsid (or nucleic acid with protein capsid) has helical symmetry and is surrounded by an envelope containing spikes of haemagglutinin and neuraminidase. × 90 000. (Photograph by Dr. E. A. C. Follett.)

3. Roughly spherical particles, medium size, 80 to 100 nm, with an envelope which contains radially-projecting spikes of virus haemagglutinin and neuraminidase; inside the envelope is a helically coiled nucleocapsid consisting of nucleoprotein, i.e. RNA surrounded by protein capsomeres (Fig. 4.1)
4. Haemagglutinate erythrocytes of various animal species
5. Grow in monkey kidney tissue culture without CPE but with haemadsorption
6. Grow in amniotic cavity of the chick embryo and—after passage or subculture—in the allantoic cavity also.

HAEMAGGLUTINATION BY INFLUENZA VIRUSES

Haemagglutination is seen with many viruses but has been most studied with influenza virus: it is due to adsorption of influenza virus particles to specific receptors on the erythrocyte surface.

Receptors are composed of sialic acid, a muco-polysaccharide—neuraminic acid.

Virus haemagglutinin is contained in the envelope round the virus particle; the haemagglutinin has a combining site which is antigenic and has an affinity for neuraminic acid.

Neuraminidase. Influenza virus particles also contain an enzyme which is similar in action to the receptor destroying enzyme (RDE) of *Vibrio cholerae*; this destroys the neuraminic receptors on erythrocytes. After viral haemagglutination, if the mixture of virus and erythrocytes is kept at 37°C, the neuraminidase becomes active and causes the virus to elute from the erythrocytes; as a result the haemagglutination is reversed and the erythrocytes disperse again.

Haemagglutination-inhibition. Treatment of the virus with specific antibody prevents haemagglutination. Haemagglutination-inhibition is strain-specific, i.e. haemagglutination by a new virus strain is unaffected by antibody to an influenza virus strain with a different haemagglutinin.

ANTIGENIC STRUCTURE

Influenza viruses have three main antigens:

1. 'S' or *soluble antigen*—the protein in the ribonucleoprotein core of the virus particle: all influenza A viruses share a common

S antigen which is different from that shared by all influenza B viruses; demonstrated by complement fixation test.

2. *Haemagglutinin*: contained in the radially-projecting spikes in the virus envelope; strain-specific; the main neutralizing antigen responsible for immunity to the virus.

3. *Neuraminidase*: also antigenic and contained in the virus envelope; plays a minor role in immunity to reinfection.

Antigenic variation

Influenza viruses are unique among viruses in that they undergo antigenic change from time to time. Epidemics are due to the emergence of a new virus strain containing a haemagglutinin (and sometimes a neuraminidase also) different from those of previously circulating viruses so that the population has no herd immunity (i.e. antibody) to the new haemagglutinin.

Antigenic variation may be:

major—*antigenic shift*
minor—*antigenic drift.*

Antigenic shift: involves the replacement of the neutralizing antigen—the haemagglutinin—by a different haemagglutinin protein acquired as a result of genetic reassortment: the appropriate RNA segment which codes for the haemagglutinin is exchanged in one virus genome for another from a different, possibly animal, virus strain. This can take place when two different influenza viruses infect and replicate in the same cell.

Antigenic shift is seen with the serological types of haemagglutinin and neuraminidase contained in the major influenza virus A strains which have circulated in the world during the past 70 years or so:

Year of emergence	Haemagglutinin	Neuraminidase
1918	H1	N1
1957	H2	N2
1968	H3	N2

Several pandemics of influenza have been recorded this century:

1. 1918–19: almost certainly due to a virus of which the haemagglutinin was similar to one commonly found in swine influenza strains
2. 1933: the first influenza virus was isolated
3. 1957: H2N2—the 'Asian flu' epidemic

4. 1968: H3N2—the 'Hong Kong flu' epidemic
5. 1977: H1N1 reappeared—'Red flu'—but caused infection only in young people under 20 years of age—because older people had antibody from exposure to the virus before 1957.

At present: both H3N2 and H1N1 strains have circulated together in countries throughout the world since 1977 (but there has been considerable antigenic drift, particularly with H3N2).

H3N2: caused a widespread epidemic in the UK in late 1989 after many years of low influenza activity: H1N1 was not isolated at this time.

Antigenic drift is due to minor changes in the amino acid sequence of the haemagglutinin protein (but the haemagglutinin basically remains the same protein). The changes are the result of spontaneous mutations; the mutant strain of virus becomes selected in the population by its ability to infect partially immune hosts: antigenic drift increases progressively from season to season.

Influenza B: also shows antigenic variation but the changes are less dramatic than with influenza A.

1. 1973: a new strain B/Hong Kong/5/73 appeared
2. 1979: B/Singapore/222/79 appeared
3. 1988: B/Yamagata/16/88 appeared.

At present: The B/Yamagata/16/88 strain shows considerable antigenic drift from the B viruses circulating in the UK in 1988; it caused widespread outbreaks in the Far East in 1989 and some infection in the USA.

Diagnosis

Serology (the most widely used)

Complement fixation test: with the 'S' or soluble antigen.

Isolation

Specimen: naso-pharyngeal aspirates are best—otherwise mouth washings or throat swabs.

Inoculate

1. Monkey kidney tissue cultures

(i) *Observe* for haemagglutination or haemadsorption of human group O erythrocytes

(ii) *Virus is typed* by haemagglutination-inhibition with specific antisera.

2. Amniotic cavity of chick embryo (now, rarely used)

(i) *Observe* for haemagglutination of fowl erythrocytes

(ii) *Virus is typed* by testing for inhibition of haemagglutination with standard antisera.

Direct demonstration

Specimen: naso-pharyngeal aspirate.

Detect virus antigen by indirect immunofluorescence.

Vaccines

At the time of a pandemic, the speed with which new strains of influenza virus spread makes it difficult if not impossible to prepare sufficient quantities of vaccine in time to protect any but a few key workers.

Virus vaccines

Contain: inactivated virus grown in fertile eggs; either purified subunits (i.e. surface antigen) or disrupted virus purified and ether-treated to solubilize envelope proteins.

Current vaccine: contains 3 strains:
influenza A, H1N1 and H3N2
influenza B, B/Yamagata/16/88.

Administered: subcutaneously.

Protection: relatively short-lived (around a few months): effective but not solid immunity (60–90% protection conferred).

Contraindicated: in people allergic to egg protein.

Guillain-Barré syndrome: a polyneuritis with ascending paralysis usually starting in the legs is a rare complication of influenza vaccine: clears up spontaneously although positive pressure respiration may be required during the acute phase due to paralysis of the respiratory muscles.

Live attenuated virus vaccines

Administered intranasally: not yet generally accepted.

5 Other respiratory tract infections

Most respiratory viruses infect both upper and lower respiratory tracts—often simultaneously. Predominantly upper respiratory syndromes usually show some involvement of the lower respiratory tract and vice versa. This chapter describes the viruses—with the exception of influenza virus—which cause respiratory disease.

Respiratory infections are a major problem in medicine because of their frequency, and are of considerable economic importance because they cause so much absence from work. So far, there is no foreseeable prospect of controlling these infections.

Spread: generally rapid and by inhalation of respiratory secretions.

Table 5.1 Viruses which affect the respiratory tract

Virus	No. of serotypes	Disease
Parainfluenza viruses	4	croup; colds, lower respiratory infections in children
Respiratory syncytial virus	1	bronchiolitis and pneumonia in infants, colds in older children
Rhinoviruses	100+	colds
Adenoviruses	41	pharyngitis and conjunctivitis
Coronaviruses	3	colds
Coxsackieviruses	types A21, B3	colds
Echoviruses	types 11, 20	colds

Infectiousness: high; most of the viruses are extremely contagious.

The principal viruses which primarily affect the respiratory tract are shown in Table 5.1.

PARAINFLUENZA VIRUSES

Clinical features

Common cold: with coryza, sore throat, hoarseness and cough and, sometimes, fever.

Croup or acute laryngo-tracheobronchitis: characterized by hoarseness, cough and inspiratory stridor in infants, the disease may be severe with respiratory distress, marked stridor and cyanosis requiring tracheostomy.

Bronchiolitis and pneumonia in young children are also sometimes caused by parainfluenza viruses.

Age. Both children and adults but infection is most common in children under 5 years old; the more severe respiratory tract infections are seen mainly in pre-school children.

Serotypes. There are four parainfluenza viruses—types 1, 2, 3 and 4—but type 4 is of lower pathogenicity.

Serotypes and disease. Although there is considerable overlap, type 3 virus is particularly associated with bronchiolitis and bronchopneumonia and types 1 and 2 with croup. Type 3 infects younger children than types 1 and 2.

Epidemiology. Parainfluenza viruses cause disease all year round but type 3 causes outbreaks of infection every year in the summer and autumn; type 1 and type 2 outbreaks are less frequent—usually every 2 years.

Immunity is not long-lasting and reinfections are common.

Virology

1. Paramyxoviruses
2. RNA viruses—single-stranded, negative sense RNA
3. Large enveloped particles, 100 to 200 nm, with helical symmetry possessing both a haemagglutinin and a neuraminidase

4. Haemagglutinate human group O erythrocytes
5. Grow in monkey kidney tissue cultures with haemadsorption.

Diagnosis

Isolation

Specimens: mouth washings, throat swabs.

Inoculate: monkey kidney tissue cultures.

Observe: for haemadsorption with human group O erythrocytes (CPE is variable and slow) or immunofluorescence.

Type virus: by neutralization test of haemadsorption by standard antisera.

Direct demonstration of virus in nasopharyngeal aspirates by immunofluorescence: a rapid technique but not yet generally available.

Serology: of limited value.

RESPIRATORY SYNCYTIAL VIRUS

Respiratory syncytial virus causes common colds but its importance lies in its tendency to invade the lower respiratory tract in infants under 1 year old causing bronchiolitis or pneumonia.

Clinical features

Colds: are the most common manifestation of infection: usually seen in children, especially in those under 5 years of age but sometimes infect the elderly in whom they can be followed by more severe lower respiratory involvement.

Bronchiolitis is a common form of disease in infants—especially in the first six months of life: the infection usually starts with nasal obstruction and discharge followed by fever, cough, rapid breathing, expiratory wheezes and signs of respiratory distress such as cyanosis and inspiratory indrawing of the intercostal spaces.

Pneumonia: also mainly seen in small infants: in respiratory syncytial virus pneumonia there is a clinical picture similar to that of bronchiolitis with fever, cyanosis, prostration and rapid breathing but without expiratory wheezing.

Bronchiolitis and pneumonia are severe diseases with a mortality rate of from 2–5%

Immunopathology. Inactivated vaccine against this virus enhanced the incidence of bronchiolitis and pneumonia in vaccinees compared to controls; since the diseases appear mainly in infants in whom maternal antibody is still present, it seemed possible that both diseases might be partly *immunological,* due to the formation of immune complexes. Alternatively, the susceptibility of very young infants to these diseases may be *mechanical* and caused by the narrowness of the bronchiolar lumen: when this is inflamed, serious obstruction may be produced more readily than in older infants with wider bronchioles. This second explanation is now the more widely accepted.

Epidemiology

Every year there are outbreaks of respiratory syncytial virus, most often during the later winter months from February to April.

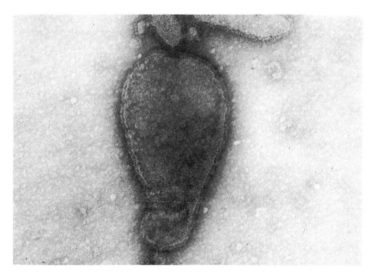

Fig. 5.1 Respiratory syncytial virus. Pleomorphic virus with helical nucleocapsid surrounded by an envelope. × 90 000. (Photograph by Dr E. A. C. Follett.)

Virology

1. Pneumovirus—within the paramyxovirus family, one serological type
2. RNA virus—single-stranded, negative sense RNA
3. Pleomorphic enveloped particles, medium size, 90 to 130 nm; helical symmetry (Fig. 5.1)
4. Grows in cells with syncytial CPE
5. Does not haemagglutinate.

Diagnosis

Direct demonstration of virus in nasopharyngeal aspirates by immunofluorescence using monoclonal antibody.

Isolation

Specimens: mouth washings, nasal secretions (not frozen during delivery because the virus is inactivated by freezing).

Inoculate: HeLa cells (Bristol strain), HEp-2 cells.

Observe: for characteristic CPE of syncytia of multinucleated giant cells.

Type virus: by immunofluorescence or by complement fixation test with standard antiserum.

Serology: complement fixation test.

RHINOVIRUSES

Rhinoviruses are the major cause of common colds.

Clinical features

Incubation period: 2 to 4 days.

Signs and symptoms. Nasal discharge with nasal obstruction, sneezing, sore throat and cough; about half the patients are mildly febrile; hoarseness and headache are common especially in adults.

Duration. On average symptoms subside in about a week but are prolonged for up to 2 weeks in a proportion of cases; complications include sinusitis and otitis media.

Spread is most common in the home or in school: rhinoviruses can also spread by contact (i.e. from hand to nose) as well as by inhalation of respiratory secretions: rhinoviruses can survive for some hours on skin or other surfaces.

Age. Infections are most frequent in pre-school children; thereafter the attack rate falls but infections are common even amongst adults.

Incidence. The reported attack rate for rhinovirus infection varies in different reports but on average the attack rate is about 0.7 rhinovirus infections per person per year.

Seasonal prevalence. Infections are found all year round but the prevalence is highest in autumn and spring.

Immunity. Neutralizing antibody is formed after rhinovirus infection both in blood and in respiratory secretions: respiratory IgA shows the main protective effect against re-infection with the particular serotype responsible: the large number of serotypes, however, gives opportunity for frequent (new) infections.

Epidemiology

This is complex as would be expected from the numerous virus serotypes. In any community at a given time, several serotypes can be found circulating; over a period of time, however, there is a gradual change in the serotypes present, probably due to increasing immunity within the population to earlier serotypes.

Virology

1. Picornaviruses (pico = small + RNA); more than 100 serotypes (there is some evidence that rhinoviruses may undergo antigenic variation)
2. RNA viruses, single-stranded, positive sense RNA
3. Small, icosahedral particles, 22 to 30 nm
4. Inactivated at acid pH (unlike the enteroviruses—the other members of the picornavirus group)
5. Grow in tissue cultures but at 33°C, instead of the usual 37°C (the temperature of the nostrils is 33°C)
6. Two groups of viruses:
   a. Most rhinoviruses (sometimes called 'H' viruses) grow only in human embryo cells—where they produce a CPE

b. 'M' rhinoviruses grow in monkey kidney as well as human embryo cells—also with CPE.

Diagnosis

Isolation

Specimens: nasal secretions, mouth washings.

Inoculate: human embryo lung and monkey kidney cell cultures.

Observe: for CPE.

Type virus: by neutralization with standard antisera.

Serology: impractical because of the large number of serological types of rhinovirus.

Note: culture of colds for rhinoviruses is not routinely carried out in virus laboratories and it is rare for isolates to be typed. This is a pity, as it has hampered epidemiological research.

ADENOVIRUSES

Respiratory infection

Clinical features

Clinically, the main symptoms of adenovirus respiratory infection are *pharyngitis* and *conjunctivitis*. The main syndromes are classified as shown in Table 5.2.

1. *Epidemic infection*: common in recruit camps where attack rates of 70% have been reported; also seen in children's institutions due to crowding together of susceptible young hosts.

2. *Endemic infection*: adenovirus infections are endemic but at a low level in the general population: they usually constitute less than 5% of the respiratory infections in the community at large; types 1, 2, 5 and 6 are associated with endemic infection, but cases of infection due to types 3 and 7 are common in the community and tend to be found in clusters.

3. *Epidemic kerato-conjunctivitis*: a form of eye infection which is spread mainly by contaminated instruments at eye clinics and surgeries; epidemics are seen in eye patients and also in shipyard and metal workers who are prone to minor eye injuries which

Table 5.2 Respiratory syndromes associated with adenoviruses

Syndrome	Adenovirus types
1. *Epidemic infection* pharyngo-conjunctival fever, acute respiratory disease	3, 4, 7, 14, 21
2. *Endemic infection* pharyngitis, follicular conjunctivitis	1, 2, 3, 5, 6, 7
3. *Epidemic kerato-conjunctivitis or 'shipyard eye'*	8, 19, 37

require treatment at eye clinics: unlike the other forms of adeno-virus disease, this disease is mainly associated with adenovirus type 8.

Faecal adenoviruses: adenoviruses are often found in the intestine—sometimes in association with respiratory infection. They can cause viral gastroenteritis and this is particularly associated with types 40 and 41 which are 'fastidious' and do not grow in routine cell cultures (see Ch. 7).

Other syndromes

Alimentary tract: faecal adenoviruses may play a role in mesenteric adenitis and possibly intussusception in children.

Bone marrow transplantation: adenovirus infection—mostly enteric—is common in recipients of these transplants.

Persistent infection: adenoviruses have a tendency to persist for long periods in tissues such as the tonsils, adenoids and, less often, kidneys: this may not be true latency but rather a low grade chronic infection.

Oncogenic properties: several adenoviruses cause cancer on injection into hamsters; the most highly oncogenic are types 12, 18 and 31. However, adenoviruses do not cause tumours in man.

Virology

1. 41 serological types which react independently in neutralization tests but share a common group complement fixing antigen

2. DNA viruses
3. Medium size: 60 to 70 nm; icosahedron-shaped particles with cubic symmetry and with fibres topped with knobs projecting from the vertices (Fig. 5.2)
4. Most haemagglutinate
5. Grow slowly in tissue cultures, (human embryonic cells or HeLa cells are best) with CPE of clusters of rounded and 'ballooned' cells.

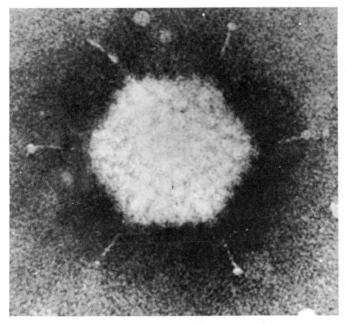

Fig. 5.2   Adenovirus. Icosahedron particle with cubic symmetry and fibres which project from the vertices. × 200 000. (Reproduced, with permission, from Valentine R. C., Pereira H. G. 1965 *Journal of Molecular Biology* 13:13.)

Diagnosis

Isolation

Specimens: mouth washings, throat swabs, faeces.

Inoculate: human embryonic cell cultures or HeLa cells.

Observe: for characteristic CPE of large rounded cells arranged like 'bunches of grapes'.

Type virus by neutralization test.

Serology: complement fixation test detects antibody to adenovirus group antigen but not the serotype of the adenovirus responsible.

OTHER VIRUSES CAUSING COMMON COLDS

Coronaviruses

Medium sized (80 to 100 nm) RNA single-stranded, positive sense viruses; characteristic enveloped particles surrounded by a fringe of club-shaped projections; haemagglutinate: can only be isolated in organ cultures of human embryo trachea although some strains, notably 229E, have been adapted to growth in the L 132 line of human embryo lung cells with CPE. There are at least 3 antigenic types although with some antigenic cross-reactions or sharing between the types.

Coronaviruses have been reported to cause as many as 30% of colds in the community but the difficulty of isolating them in the laboratory means that they are seldom diagnosed.

Enteroviruses

Some enteroviruses cause respiratory infections; the main types associated with respiratory disease are coxsackievirus A21 (formerly called Coe virus), B3 and echovirus types 11 and 20).

6 Neurological disease due to viruses

Neurological disease is a serious and not uncommon complication of virus infection. Most human pathogenic viruses are capable of spreading to the central nervous system (CNS).

Virus lesions in the CNS are due mainly to *viral multiplication* in the cells of the nervous tissue with cellular damage and dysfunction and consequent neurological signs and symptoms. But the *immune response of the host* also seems to play a role in causing lesions. In one form of viral CNS disease (post-infectious encephalomyelitis) virus cannot be isolated from the CNS.

Spread: most viruses invade the CNS by the *blood stream* but some, e.g. rabies, reach the CNS by the *neural route* by spread along the peripheral nerves.

CNS involvement is not always followed by neurological disease—for example there is evidence that symptomless involvement of the CNS is common in measles and mumps.

Virus neurological diseases fall into two clinical categories—acute and chronic.

ACUTE VIRAL NEUROLOGICAL DISEASE

There are four main syndromes:

1. *Encephalitis.* The main symptoms are drowsiness, mental confusion, convulsions, focal neurological signs and sometimes coma
2. *Paralysis.* With fever, flaccid paralysis—most often of the lower limbs—and signs of meningitis such as headache with stiffness of neck and back
3. *Aseptic meningitis.* A relatively mild disease with fever, headache and stiffness of neck and back

Table 6.1 Acute virus neurological diseases

	Direct invasion of CNS by virus			Virus not demonstrable in CNS (disease is probably due to abnormal immune response of host to infection)
Disease	Encephalitis	Paralysis (poliomyelitis)	Aseptic meningitis	Post-infectious encephalomyelitis
Site	Brain	Anterior horn cells of spinal cord	Meninges	Brain
Lesions	Destructive lesions in grey matter; neuronal damage	Destructive lesions of lower motor neurones with meningitis	Inflammation of meninges, cells in CSF (usually lymphocytes)	Perivascular infiltration, microglial proliferation, demyelination
Viruses	Herpes simplex, arboviruses rabies	Enteroviruses (especially polioviruses)	Enteroviruses, mumps, lymphocytic choriomeningitis	Measles, rubella, varicella-zoster, vaccinia

Table 6.2 Chronic virus neurological diseases

Disease	Subacute sclerosing panencephalitis	Progressive multifocal leucoencephalopathy	Creutzfeldt-Jakob disease	Kuru
Site	Brain	Brain	Brain and spinal cord	Brain
Lesions	Neuronal degeneration, intranuclear inclusions	Multiple foci of degeneration	Spongiform degeneration	Spongiform degeneration especially in cerebellum
Viruses	Measles, rubella (after congenital infection)	JC virus	Transmissible by filter-passing agent	Transmissible by filter-passing agent

4. *Post-infectious encephalomyelitis* (also called encephalitis). Symptoms are similar to those of encephalitis.

Table 6.1 summarizes the principal features of the four main acute viral neurological syndromes.

CHRONIC VIRUS NEUROLOGICAL DISEASES

Viruses cause several chronic neurological diseases which are listed in Table 6.2 and which are described in more detail in Chapter 16. Below are listed some of the main features:

1. *Rare.* All the diseases are very rare and most doctors will never see a case of any of them throughout their working lives.
2. *Signs and symptoms.* Numerous and varied: neurological and often affect intellectual capacity as well as both motor and sensory functions
3. *Duration.* The diseases may last for months or even years but are relentlessly progressive
4. *Fatal.* The diseases are always fatal.

7 Enterovirus infections

Enteroviruses are a large family of viruses, of which the primary site of infection is the gut; nevertheless, they rarely cause intestinal symptoms; enterovirus diseases are the result of spread of the viruses to other sites of the body—particularly the CNS.

Below are listed the various groups included in the enterovirus family:

		Enteroviruses			
		coxsackieviruses*		echoviruses†	enteroviruses (unclassified)
		group A	group B		
Types	1-3	1-24	1-6	1-34	68-72‡

* Coxsackie is the village in New York where these viruses were first isolated:
† Enteric, Cytopathic, Human, Orphan (Orphan because originally—but wrongly—thought not to be associated with human disease).
‡ Enterovirus 72 was Hepatitis A virus (see Ch. 14) but this virus has now been reclassified

Enteroviruses have the following properties:

Enter the body via ingestion by mouth.

Primary site of multiplication is the lymphoid tissue of the alimentary tract—including the pharynx.

Spread from the gut is in two directions:

1. *Outwards* into the blood (viraemia) and so to other tissues and organs
2. *Inwards* into the lumen of the gut and to excretion into the faeces.

Clinical features

The main enterovirus diseases are shown in Table 7.1.

Table 7.1 Enterovirus disease

Syndrome	Main viruses responsible
1. Neurological	
(i) Paralysis	(i) polioviruses
(ii) Aseptic meningitis	(ii) most enteroviruses
2. Febrile illness	most enteroviruses
3. Herpangina; hand, foot and mouth disease	coxsackie A viruses
4. Myocarditis, pericarditis	coxsackie B viruses
5. Bornholm disease	coxsackie B viruses
6. Acute haemorrhagic conjunctivitis	enterovirus 70

General features of enterovirus infections: most infections are confined to the alimentary tract and are symptomless: enteroviruses do not cause diarrhoea.

A small proportion of infections give rise to febrile illness due to viraemia.

Still fewer cases progress to aseptic meningitis and—more rarely still—to paralysis: spread of virus to the CNS or other organs and tissues is a rare complication of enterovirus infection.

NEUROLOGICAL SYNDROMES

Neurological disease is nevertheless the most important manifestation of enteroviral infection; it is not associated with one particular group or type of enterovirus—although some enteroviruses are more prone to cause neurological symptoms than others.

The illness is usually biphasic: the initial symptoms are of febrile illness due to viraemia; there is an intervening period of well-being for a day or two followed by the onset of neurological symptoms; these are due to spread of the virus through the 'blood-brain barrier' to invade the CNS.

There are two main types of neurological syndrome due to enteroviruses:

1. *Paralysis* or poliomyelitis: an acute illness with pain and *flaccid* paralysis affecting mainly the lower legs. Sometimes the muscles of respiration become involved requiring tracheostomy with artificial ventilation: more rarely, the disease may take the form of *bulbar paralysis* when the muscles of breathing and swallowing are primarily involved. Paralysis is an extension of aseptic meningitis and is therefore accompanied by the signs and symptoms of that syndrome.

Pathology: paralysis is due to viral damage to the cells of the anterior horn of the spinal cord with lower motor neurone lesions resulting in flaccid paralysis. If damage to the nerve cells is severe, the paralysis becomes irreversible (Plate 1).

Paralysis is most often due to the three polioviruses and especially poliovirus 1. Before the introduction of poliovaccine, epidemics of paralysis were common in countries with a high standard of living e.g. USA, Denmark, Australia.

2. *Aseptic meningitis*: is much more common than paralysis; although signs of CNS disease are present, the damage is minor; the main features are fever and headache with nuchal rigidity (stiffness of the neck muscles due to meningeal irritation). Lymphocytes and protein in the cerebrospinal fluid (CSF) are increased. The prognosis is good and most patients recover completely.

NON-NEUROLOGICAL SYNDROMES

Febrile illness: a common manifestation of any enterovirus infection and due to viraemia.

Rash: many enteroviruses cause rash but this is particularly common with coxsackie A9 and A16 (see below) and echovirus 9.

Herpangina: a painful eruption of vesicles in the mouth and throat: recently, it has been reported as part of the syndrome of 'hand, foot and mouth disease' in which there are also vesicles on the hand and feet; due to group A coxsackieviruses (especially A16); enterovirus 71 has also caused hand, foot and mouth disease.

Bornholm disease: also known as pleurodynia or epidemic myalgia: a painful inflammation of muscles which mainly involves the intercostal muscles. The disease is named after the Danish island where there was an extensive outbreak in 1930; due to group B coxsackieviruses.

Myocarditis and pericarditis: due to group B coxsackieviruses. *Myocarditis* is characterized by rapid pulse, enlargement of the heart and ECG abnormalities and pericarditis by pericardial friction or effusion.

Either syndrome can be present on its own but patients often develop myocarditis and pericarditis together. Both diseases are seen mainly in adult males, and may be mistaken for myocardial infarction; however, the prognosis is good and most patients recover completely. Rarely, epidemics have been reported among neonates in hospital nurseries. In the 1965 epidemic of coxsackievirus B5 infections in England and Wales, 15% of the patients had cardiac signs or symptoms, the incidence being higher in adults than in children.

Acute haemorrhagic conjunctivitis: due to enterovirus 70 has appeared in large-scale outbreaks in 1969–71 in Africa, South-East Asia, Japan, India and, although to a limited extent, in Britain. The incubation period is 24 hours and the disease lasts about 10 days: patients recover completely: the disease spreads rapidly, probably via eye discharges. Unlike most enterovirus infections the causal virus is not found in the faeces.

Epidemiology

Enterovirus infections are common—especially in children and in conditions of poor hygiene. In children in tropical or developing countries, multiple infection of the gut with several different viruses simultaneously is common.

Infection is spread mainly by the faecal-oral route from virus excretors to contacts; virus in pharyngeal secretions may also be a source of infection.

Gut immunity: after infection with an enterovirus, the gut becomes resistant to reinfection with the same virus; this resistance is due to the production in the gut of virus-specific neutralizing IgA antibody.

Seasonal distribution: infections are much more frequent in the summer than in the winter months.

Epidemics of aseptic meningitis used to be common with one or sometimes two viruses predominating. Nowadays the epidemiology is more of sporadic infections, which increase in incidence during the summer months, and with several different viruses responsible. In the past, epidemics were often associated with echovirus 9 and, before widespread use of poliovaccine, with polioviruses; echoviruses 4, 6, 11, 14, 16 and 30 and coxsackieviruses A9 and B5 have also caused epidemic aseptic meningitis.

Poor sanitation, e.g. in developing countries, increases the chances of childhood infection so that immunity is acquired in childhood.

High standard of living in countries such as the USA, diminishes the chance of infection and therefore of immunity being acquired in childhood.

Adults are more liable to develop severe paralysis in poliovirus infection than children: the risk of this is increased by pregnancy, tonsillectomy, fatigue, trauma or inoculation with bacterial vaccines.

Epidemics: countries with a high standard of living have a relatively large proportion of non-immune adults and before the advent of poliovaccines suffered from repeated and widespread epidemics of paralytic disease.

Virology

1. Picornaviruses (pico = small + RNA)
2. RNA viruses, single-stranded, positive sense RNA
3. Small roughly spherical particles, 25 to 30 nm (Fig. 7.1)
4. Stable at acid pH (in contrast to the rhinoviruses—the other members of the picornavirus group)
5. Most grow in tissue cultures with rapid CPE
6. Coxsackieviruses (but not polio or echoviruses) are pathogenic for suckling mice.

Diagnosis

Isolation

Specimens: faeces, throat swabs: CSF is useful for some viruses (e.g. echovirus 9) but not for polioviruses.

Inoculate: monkey kidney, human embryo lung cell cultures.

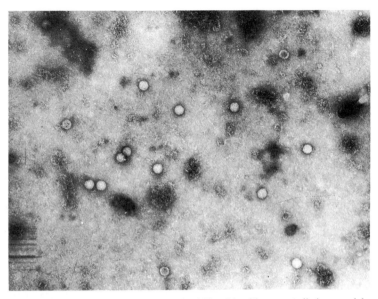

Fig. 7.1   Echovirus. All enteroviruses look like this with very small virus particles with cubic symmetry.' × 90 000. (Photograph by Dr E. A. C. Follett.)

Observe: for CPE.

Type virus: by neutralization tests with standard antisera; usually done using pools of antisera to reduce the number of tests.

Note: Most coxsackie A viruses do not grow in tissue cultures so if coxsackie A virus infection is suspected:

(i) *Inoculate*: suckling mice subcutaneously and intracerebrally
(ii) *Observe*: for characteristic signs of disease—group A coxsackieviruses cause flaccid paralysis due to widespread myositis.

Note: Group B coxsackieviruses cause spastic paralysis with tremor due to cerebral lesions and fat-pad necrosis.

Serology

Neutralization tests are useful for the diagnosis of poliomyelitis.

ELISA tests can be used to detect IgM to group B coxsackieviruses.

Apart from this, the large number of enteroviruses makes serological diagnosis impracticable.

Vaccination

Two vaccines are available against the three polioviruses.

1. **Sabin live attenuated virus vaccine.** Now the main vaccine used for the poliomyelitis immunization.

Contains the three polioviruses as attenuated strains which have lost neurovirulence for monkeys (i.e. ability to produce paralysis or lesions in CNS of monkeys); grown in monkey kidney tissue cultures.

Administered in three oral doses along with triple vaccine starting at 2 months of age and with an interval of 1 month between each dose: boosters at school entry and when leaving school.

Protection: good.

Blood antibody response: good.

Gut immunity: good; vaccinated children show increased resistance to alimentary infection; this is due to the appearance of virus-specific IgA in the gut produced in response to the vaccine.

Safety: good; very rarely paralysis—usually mild and usually due to the type 3 component: incidence about 1 per million doses.

Vaccinated children are infectious to others so that vaccine strains may circulate to some extent in the community.

Widespread use of this vaccine has resulted in a dramatic decrease both in paralytic poliomyelitis and in the circulation of wild polioviruses in the community.

2. **Salk inactivated virus vaccine.** This was the first polio vaccine to be used on a large scale but is now less widely used than Sabin vaccine. It contains the three polioviruses inactivated by formaldehyde and is given in three injections. Although producing good blood antibody levels—and therefore good protection against paralysis—it fails to give gut immunity. Nevertheless, modern Salk vaccine is of improved, high potency and is used successfully in Scandinavia. There is at present discussion in the UK as to whether the primary course of the polio vaccine should be Salk vaccine with later booster of Sabin vaccine.

8 Viral gastroenteritis

Viruses are an important cause of acute diarrhoea—most often, but not exclusively in young children. In developing countries viral gastroenteritis plays a major role in the high infant mortality, although in Britain the disease is now generally mild. Several viruses are responsible, but because they are fastidious and do not grow in routine cell culture, electron microscopy has been used to detect and identify them. Nevertheless, morphology alone is a limited technique for investigation—both virological and epidemiological. For example, the ecology of these viruses, their pathogenicity—even their mode of spread and relative frequency in normal populations as well as in patients with diarrhoea—is still largely unknown. The main viruses associated with acute diarrhoea are listed in Table 8.1.

The table illustrates the main criteria for classification of the viruses—namely particle morphology. Although calicivirus, Norwalk virus and small round structured (SRSVs) and non-structured (SRVs) viruses are shown as separate groups, there is some evidence that they may in fact be closely related. Most of the virus groups listed have their counterpart in animals—both domesticated and wild. Indeed, in some cases, such as rotavirus, animal strains were discovered and investigated before the human viruses were known.

Clinical features

Incubation period: short, 1–2 days.

Symptoms: acute onset of diarrhoea, often with vomiting—which may be projectile—and sometimes with fever: abdominal cramps: dehydration—with hyponatraemia—is a common complication and requires correction with oral, sometimes, parenteral, rehydration fluids.

Table 8.1   Viruses causing diarrhoea

Virus	Nucleic acid	Particle	No. of serotypes
Rotavirus	DS RNA in 11 Segments	70 nm double-shelled with wheel-like surface structure	9
Astrovirus	SS RNA	28 nm, 6-pointed star surface structure	5
Adenovirus	DS RNA	74 nm, classical icosahedron with rounded capsomeres	2 (types 40, 41)
Calicivirus	SS RNA	33 nm, 6-pointed star surface structure with central 'hole'	4
Norwalk	SS RNA	35 nm, indistinct surface structure	Not known
Small round viruses (SRVs)	Not known	22–25 nm, small, round, featureless	Not known
Small Round structured viruses (SRSVs)	Not known	35 nm, ill-defined surface structure	Not known

Note: the number of serotypes quoted are based on current—but incomplete —knowledge

Winter vomiting disease: is a form of viral gastroenteritis in which vomiting is a much more prominent feature than diarrhoea: it tends to be associated with calicivirus or Norwalk virus.

Age: mainly affects infants aged between 6 months and 2 years, but older children and more rarely adults can also be affected.

Season: most common in the winter months.

Geographical distribution: world-wide distribution but highest incidence in conditions of poor sanitation, overcrowding and poverty.

Epidemiology

Endemic infection: is widespread.

Epidemics: or outbreaks of infection, are seen more often associated with some viruses (e.g. SRVs, Norwalk virus) than others.

Treatment

Symptomatic: rehydration with care to correct sodium loss (or hyponatraemia if rehydrating salt solutions are used too liberally).

VIRUSES

Rotavirus

The first virus to be associated with acute non-bacterial gastro-enteritis: mainly affects infants but, although it is difficult to infect adult volunteers experimentally, outbreaks have been reported in adults—most often among the elderly in hospitals or residential homes.

Site of infection: the upper small intestine.

Pathogenicity: there is no doubt that rotavirus causes gastro-enteritis, but infection is quite commonly symptomless—and virus can be demonstrated in the stools of healthy controls. Infection in the neonate is often not accompanied with diarrhoea.

Route of infection: faecal-oral from case to case, but respiratory symptoms have been described in rotavirus infection and respiratory secretions may also be a source of spread.

Epidemiology—infection is mainly endemic, but outbreaks—several in adults—have been reported.

Virology

1. Reovirus family
2. RNA, double-stranded, in 11 fragments, which form characteristic banding patterns on electrophoresis
3. Particles—are characteristic (Fig. 8.1 and Table 8.1)
4. Five groups A–E of which groups D and E are found only in animals. Group A strains—the most common in humans— are sub-divided into two sub-groups (I and II) which contain 9 serotypes
5. Can now be grown in tissue culture, but only by special techniques.

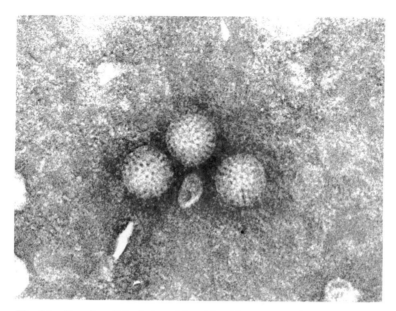

Fig. 8.1   Rotavirus. Spherical particles with cubic symmetry, showing
characteristic outer layer like the spokes of a wheel, which distinguishes the virus
from reovirus. × 200 000. (Photograph by Prof. C. R. Madeley.)

Diagnosis

Demonstration of virus in the stools by:

1. *Electron microscopy*
2. *Serology*—ELISA, latex agglutination.

Astroviruses

Found significantly more often in the stools of children with
diarrhoea than in those from healthy controls; astroviruses are
therefore clearly associated with diarrhoea. They have been
reported in several outbreaks in hospital and within families, but
only rarely outside the UK.

Virology—little is known

1. RNA virus—single-stranded RNA

2. Particles, distinguishable (but with difficulty) from those of caliciviruses which they resemble: see Table 8.1
3. Serotypes—5 have been reported.

Diagnosis

Electron microscopy of stools.

Adenovirus

Respiratory adenoviruses can also, not uncommonly, be cultured from stools. Diarrhoea-causing adenoviruses (sometimes called group F adenoviruses) are 'fastidious' and do not grow in routine cell cultures: they are serologically distinct from respiratory strains. Found in endemic infections in the community and also in outbreaks: infection is often associated with prolonged excretion.

Virology

Fastidious adenoviruses have the characteristic properties of all adenoviruses but belong to two new serotypes 40 and 41. They can now be cultivated by special techniques in cell culture.

Diagnosis

Electron microscopy of stools.

Calicivirus

Like the viruses discussed above, caliciviruses are found more often in stools of children with diarrhoea than in those from healthy controls. But they are less commonly associated with diarrhoea than astroviruses. They are found in outbreaks of vomiting and diarrhoea rather than in endemic infections. Vomiting tends to be a prominent symptom and caliciviruses have been incriminated as a major cause of outbreaks of winter vomiting disease.

Virology

1. RNA virus—single-stranded, positive sense RNA

2. Particle (see Table 8.1) can be difficult to differentiate from those of some of the other diarrhoea-associated viruses
3. Serological: there is evidence of three serotypes.

Diagnosis

Electron microscopy of stools.

Norwalk virus

Norwalk virus has been repeatedly reported as a cause of outbreaks—mainly in the USA—although the distribution of the virus is world-wide. Vomiting is a prominent symptom in Norwalk virus infections.

Virology

1. RNA virus—single-stranded, positive sense RNA
2. Particle—(see Table 8.1) similar to particles of SRSVs
3. Serology—unknown. Probably multiple types.

Diagnosis

Electron microscopy of stools.

Small round viruses—structured (SRSVs) and non-structured (SRVs)

Little is known of the characteristics, classification and epidemiology of these viruses, but they are often detected in the stools of patients involved in outbreaks. Outbreaks have been traced to raw shellfish. Such evidence as is available indicates most outbreaks are due to different serotypes of virus.

Virology

Little is known: SRVs are smaller than SRSVs of which the structure detectable on the surface of the particles is ill-defined. There is some indication that SRSVs may be different serotypes in the same virus family group as calicivirus and Norwalk virus.

VIRUS DIARRHOEA

The electron microscope has identified the many viruses that cause this important disease. But further research is needed—not only into the virology of these agents, but into their epidemiology. Progress will be slow until they can be grown in tissue culture: this has already been achieved with some and, given the advances in biotechnology, the next few years should see this accomplished with the others.

9 Arthropod-borne virus infections

Many virus diseases are transmitted by the bite of an arthropod vector. The viruses are called *arboviruses* and multiply in the bodies of arthropods.

Arboviruses are extremely numerous and include many unrelated viruses belonging to different virus groups:

1. *Alphavirus* (formerly group A arbovirus)
2. *Flavivirus* (formerly group B arbovirus)
3. *Bunyaviruses*
   Subdivided into
   a. *Bunyavirus*
   b. *Nairovirus*
   c. *Phlebovirus*
   d. *Uukuvirus*
   e. *Hantavirus* (not arthropod-borne—see Chapter 10).

Vectors: Mosquitoes, ticks and sandflies are the principal arthropod vectors which transmit arboviruses.

Animal hosts. The main reservoirs are wild birds and small mammals; the viruses spread to man when an arthropod vector acquires virus from its natural host and transmits it in the course of biting the human host.

Disease. Arboviruses cause two types of diseases:

1. Encephalitis
2. Fever (often with haemorrhage).

Some of the most important arboviruses are listed in Table 9.1 together with their vectors and the diseases they produce.

Table 9.1   Classification of arboviruses

Virus	Disease	Vector
Alphaviruses		
Eastern equine encephalitis	Encephalitis	Mosquito
Western equine encephalitis	Encephalitis	Mosquito
Venezuelan equine encephalitis	Encephalitis, febrile disease	Mosquito
Chikungunya	Febrile disease	Mosquito
Ross River	Febrile disease	Mosquito
Flaviviruses		
St Louis encephalitis	Encephalitis	Mosquito
Japanese B encephalitis	Encephalitis	Mosquito
Murray Valley encephalitis	Encephalitis	Mosquito
Tick-borne encephalitis	Encephalitis	Tick
Yellow fever	Haemorrhagic fever	Mosquito
Rocio	Encephalitis	Mosquito
Kyasanur Forest disease	Haemorrhagic fever	Tick
Omsk haemorrhagic fever	Haemorrhagic fever	Tick
Dengue	Febrile disease, haemorrhagic fever	Mosquito
Bunyaviruses		
California encephalitis	Encephalitis	Mosquito
Oropouche	Febrile disease	Midge
Nairovirus		
Crimean-Congo haemorrhagic fever	Haemorrhagic fever	Tick
Phlebovirus		
Rift Valley fever	Febrile disease, haemorrhagic fever	Mosquito
Phlebotomus fever	Febrile disease	Sandfly

ARBOVIRUS ENCEPHALITIS

Arbovirus encephalitis is a world-wide problem. It is common in North and South America (Eastern, Western and Venezuelan equine encephalitis, Rociovirus, yellow fever, California and St Louis encephalitis), Africa (Chikungunya, yellow fever), the Far East (Japanese B encephalitis), Eastern Europe (tick-borne encephalitis) and Australia (Murray Valley encephalitis). Dengue is a serious mosquito-borne infection found, often in epidemics, over large areas of Asia, Africa, the Caribbean and South America. Arboviruses are not a problem in Britain where the only virus found is that causing the tick-borne disease, louping ill, in sheep—and only occasionally in man.

Clinical features

The main symptoms are fever, progressively severe headache, nausea, vomiting, stiffness of neck, back and legs; there may be convulsions, drowsiness, deepening coma and neurological signs such as paralysis and tremor.

Symptomless infection is common with most of the arboviruses which cause encephalitis. After an epidemic, arbovirus antibodies are present in a considerable proportion of the population; the incidence of encephalitis as a result of the arbovirus infection is usually low although some viruses, e.g. Eastern equine encephalitis virus, cause symptoms in a higher proportion of people infected than others, e.g. Venezuelan equine encephalitis. Eastern equine encephalitis also has a higher mortality rate.

Age. Arbovirus encephalitis affects all ages although some variations are seen with different viruses. For example, California encephalitis is mainly seen in school children whereas St Louis encephalitis produces its most severe effects in older people in whom neurological sequelae are common; Western equine encephalitis on the other hand produces more sequelae in young people.

Epidemics of arbovirus encephalitis are common and have been well studied in the USA: epidemics are seasonal, infection being more frequent in summer and in autumn. Before and during a human epidemic there is evidence of infection spreading in the animals, e.g. birds, that are the natural hosts of the virus; in Eastern, Western and Venezuelan equine encephalitis, epidemics of human infection are preceded by, or concurrent with, epidemic infection in horses. The horses, like man, are secondary hosts of the viruses, the primary or natural hosts being birds (Eastern and Western) and small mammals (Venezuelan).

ARBOVIRUS FEVERS AND HAEMORRHAGIC FEVERS

These syndromes overlap to some extent in that haemorrhages are not infrequent complication of arbovirus fevers; there is some evidence that the haemorrhagic forms of disease may be due to formation of immune complexes due to abnormally large production of antibodies.

Note: haemorrhagic fevers are also caused by other, non-arthropod-borne viruses (see Ch. 10).

Epidemiology. Worldwide in distribution especially in semi-tropical and tropical countries; epidemics are frequent and are a major health problem. Symptomless infection—detected by a relatively high prevalence of antibodies in the general population concerned—is common.

Clinically, the symptoms are those of a severe generalized febrile disease with high fever, chills, severe headache, pain in the limbs, nausea and vomiting; some arbovirus fevers have additional signs and symptoms such as rash or arthritis.

Below are some of the best known arbovirus fevers:

Yellow fever

Yellow fever is one of the most important haemorrhagic fevers, but with liver involvement and jaundice as characteristic features. Historically, the cause of many deaths ('yellow jack') in early colonialists from Europe in Central and South America. Still a problem despite an effective vaccine and its susceptibility to mosquito control measures. Endemic in South America and the central belt of Africa. There are two forms:

1. *Urban,* in which the reservoir of the virus is man and the vector the mosquito *Aedes aegypti.*
2. *Sylvan or jungle,* in which the reservoir is tree-dwelling monkeys and the vector various species of forest mosquito.

Clinically, the most striking feature of yellow fever is jaundice due to viral involvement of the liver causing hepatitis; haemorrhages are often seen and a toxic nephrosis with proteinuria is a common feature.

Diagnosis

Serology: by haemagglutination-inhibition, neutralization or complement fixation tests.

Kyasanur Forest fever

A haemorrhagic fever which affects forest workers in Mysore State, India: the animal reservoirs are monkeys. Interestingly, the virus is widespread in India but the disease is seen only in Mysore State.

Dengue

A major health problem in South-east Asia, India, the Pacific Islands, and the Caribbean; infection is widespread in these areas; monkeys are probably the main reservoir of infection and the main vector is *Aedes aegypti*.

Antigenic types: there are four sub-types (types 1 to 4) of dengue virus.

Clinically, dengue typically presents as a severe febrile disease with pain in the limbs and rash; the case fatality rate of this type of dengue is low.

Dengue haemorrhagic shock syndrome: a serious complication of dengue in young children. In this syndrome, an attack of dengue progresses to a more severe disease characterized by haemorrhages and shock; seen in children who have experienced a previous attack of dengue due to a different sub-type of virus: on re-infection with the second virus, immune complexes are formed due to production of excess antibody; the immune complexes with complement activation are responsible for the haemorrhagic shock syndrome.

Chikunguna

The cause of febrile disease—sometimes in widespread epidemics —in Africa and Asia. In Asia the disease has had haemorrhagic manifestations.

Clinically, characterized by sudden fever with severe pain in the joints. Residual joint pains may persist after recovery from the acute disease.

O'nyong-nyong: due to a similar virus is a febrile disease with joint pain (the name means 'break-bone fever'): seen in Africa in small outbreaks but there was a large epidemic in 1959–60.

Ross River virus

The cause of epidemics in Australia and the Pacific of febrile disease with rash and polyarthritis.

Congo/Crimean haemorrhagic fever

This severe disease is seen in southern Russia, Bulgaria, central and southern Africa, the Middle East and Pakistan: can also spread case-to-case to medical and nursing staff via contact with infected blood.

Clinically, the disease has a high mortality rate: the most serious cases show a marked haemorrhagic tendency sometimes with extensive skin ecchymoses and circulatory collapse. There is evidence that severely haemorrhagic cases have a greater antibody response than patients with milder disease.

Oropouche

This bunyavirus has caused epidemics of febrile disease in Brazil, with headaches, myalgia, joint pains and sometimes neurological involvement such as meningitis or even encephalitis.

Rift Valley fever

Responsible for large epizootics in sheep and cattle in Africa—particularly Egypt, the Sudan and South Africa. Human infection is acquired through contact with infected animals as well as via mosquito bite. The human disease is a febrile disease with headache, nausea, vomiting and haemorrhages in severe cases: some patients have developed retinitis.

Virology

The following are some properties of the main arbovirus groups:

Alphaviruses

1. 25 recognized viruses
2. RNA viruses—single-stranded, positive sense RNA
3. Enveloped particles, roughly spherical, about 70 nm in diameter (Fig. 9.1)

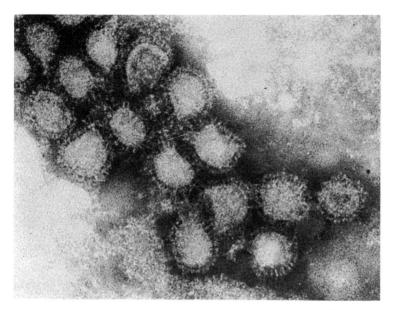

Fig. 9.1   An alphavirus. This photograph of sindbis virus shows roughly spherical particles with cubic symmetry and a surface fringe. × 200 000. (Photograph by Prof. C. R. Madeley.)

4. Haemagglutinate avian red cells
5. Grow in cell culture: pathogenic for suckling mice.

Flaviviruses

1. 60 viruses
2. RNA viruses—single-stranded, positive sense RNA
3. Enveloped particles—from 40–50 nm in diameter
4. Haemagglutinate avian red cells
5. Grow in cell culture: pathogenic for suckling mice.

Bunyaviruses

1. A large family containing 150 viruses in 6 genera (see p.77).
2. RNA viruses—single-stranded, negative sense RNA in three segments, thus giving opportunity for genetic reassortment
3. Enveloped particles, approximately 90–100 nm in diameter
4. Haemagglutinate

5. Grow in cell culture: generally pathogenic for suckling mice or other rodents.

Diagnosis of arbovirus infection

Complex, requires facilities of specialist, reference laboratories. Generally by

1. Serology (complement fixation, haemagglutination-inhibition, neutralization)
2. Isolation from blood (e.g. throat swab, CSF etc) by inoculation of:
  (i) suckling mice
  (ii) cell culture (where appropriate).

Vaccines

The most widely used vaccine available for arboviruses is against yellow fever but effective vaccines are also available for Japanese and tick-borne encephalitis, and on a limited basis for those at special risk, for Eastern, Western and Venezuelan equine encephalitis. Vaccines against dengue are being developed.

Yellow fever vaccine

Contains live attenuated virus of a strain known as 17D attenuated by repeated passage in chick embryos.

Prepared in chick embryos.

Administered in one dose by subcutaneous injection.

Protection conferred is good, solid immunity which lasts for at least 10 years.

Safety: good, singularly free from side-effects.

10 Rabies, non-arthropod-borne haemorrhagic fevers, arenavirus infections

The diseases to be described in this chapter are zoonoses, i.e. they are acquired from animals which are reservoirs of infection.

RABIES

Rabies is a lethal form of encephalitis due to a virus which affects a wide variety of animal species: rabies is transmitted to man via the bite of an infected animal which is usually—but not always—a dog.

Clinical features

The incubation period is long—usually from 4 to 12 weeks but sometimes much longer and occasionally more than a year; if the wound is on the head or neck the incubation period is shorter than for wounds on the limbs.

Virus spread from the wound to the CNS is via the nerves.

Symptoms: initially: paraesthesia in the wound is an early symptom. Thereafter there are two forms of rabies:

(i) *furious*: the more common of the two, in which the symptoms are excitement, with tremor, muscular contractions and convulsions; typically spasm of the muscle of swallowing (hence the older name for the disease of 'hydrophobia' or fear of water) and increased sensitivity of the sensory nervous system (Plate 2).
(ii) *dumb*: or paralytic rabies in which the symptoms are of ascending paralysis, eventually involving the muscles of swallowing, speech and respiration.

Virus is present in saliva, skin and eyes as well as the brain.

Prognosis: the disease is virtually always fatal (although there have been rare reports of recovery); death often follows a convulsion.

Pathology: despite the severity of the clinical disease, lesions in the CNS are often minimal with little evidence of destructive effects on cells; the main changes are the intracytoplasmic inclusions within neurones known as Negri bodies and diagnostic of rabies.

Epidemiology

Rabies is a natural infection of dogs, cats, bats and carnivorous wild animals such as foxes, wolves, skunks: infection is also found in rodents and cattle (especially in South America where the virus is spread by the bite of infected vampire bats). Human exposure to rabies is generally most common from dogs. In under-developed countries, infection in urban dogs poses a major problem and a risk to man.

Virus is present in the saliva of infected dogs—sometimes for up to four days before the onset of symptoms of the disease; dogs and cats which remain healthy for ten days after biting can be regarded as being free of virus at the time of biting.

Incidence of rabies after biting: relatively few—about 15%—of people bitten by a rabid animal develop the disease; rabies is more common after bites on the head or neck than after wounds on the limbs.

Britain is at present free from indigenous rabies. Rabies used to be present in animals in Britain but was eradicated by 1921; the strict six-month quarantine laws for animals imported into Britain have been successful in keeping out the disease. Smuggling of pet animals into Britain to avoid the quarantine regulations is fairly common and represents a potential source of importation of the virus. The main danger is that rabies might become established as a reservoir of infection in wild animals. If this happens, given Britain's fairly large fox population, it might prove difficult to eradicate the disease. Rabies is present in wild animals in all continents of the world with the exception of Australia (and Antartica). Most important from a British point of view is its spread as an epizootic, slowly moving westward from Eastern Europe across France.

Aerosol infection: has been recorded—as a result of laboratory accident, or acquired in bat-infested caves: a very rare event.

Case to case spread: human patients do not seem to be a source of infection to medical attendants despite the presence of virus in saliva—see below.

Corneal transplant: cases of rabies in recipients of corneas from donors of undiagnosed rabies have been reported.

Virology

1. A member of the *lyssavirus* genus within the *rhabdovirus* family: rabies is the most neurotropic of the antigenically-related group of lyssaviruses which naturally infect many different animal species.
2. RNA virus—negative sense, single-stranded RNA
3. Bullet-shaped, enveloped particles containing helically-coiled nucleoprotein; length 180 nm, diameter 70 to 80 nm (Fig. 10.1)

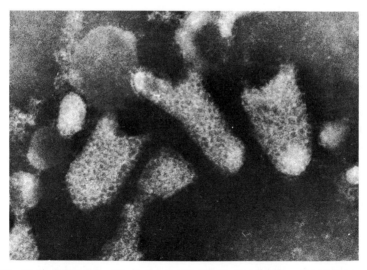

Fig. 10.1   Rabies virus. The nucleocapsid of the bullet-shaped particles has helical symmetry and is surrounded by an envelope. × 180 000. (Photograph by Prof. C. R. Madeley.)

4. Haemagglutinates goose erythrocytes
5. Grows in hamster kidney and chick embryo cell tissue cultures with eosinophilic cytoplasmic inclusions but usually without CPE
6. Pathogenic for mice and other laboratory animals.

Diagnosis

Direct demonstration of virus

Specimens: hair-bearing skin (e.g. back of neck), corneal impression smears, brain tissue.

Examine: for presence of rabies virus antigen by immunofluorescence.

Negri bodies: a less sensitive method of diagnosis: examine brain smears of the Ammon's horn of the hippocampus stained with Seller's stain for red intracytoplasmic intrusions (Negri bodies.)

Isolation

Specimens: brain tissue, saliva, CSF, urine.

Inoculate: mice intra-cerebrally.

Observe: for paralysis, convulsions; post-mortem for immunofluorescence with rabies antiserum and Negri bodies in brain cells.

Note: if rabies is suspected in a dog it should be kept under observation to see if the disease develops, and not killed right away; if it is killed before death due to the disease, Negri bodies may not have developed in sufficient numbers to be detected in histological sections. After death, the dog's head is sent to a specialist laboratory for examination.

Vaccination

Rabies vaccine was first developed by Pasteur in 1885; it consisted of virus attenuated by drying the spinal cords of infected rabbits for varying lengths of time over KOH. Wild rabies virus is known as 'street' virus and attenuated virus as 'fixed' virus. All vaccines prepared for human use contain inactivated virus.

The long incubation period makes rabies a suitable disease for prophylactic immunization after exposure.

After exposure—or suspicion of exposure—to rabies, the wound should be thoroughly washed with soap and water, alcohol, iodine solutions or quaternary ammonium compound; patients should be given combined passive and active immunization.

Passive immunization: by injection of human anti-rabies immunoglobulin.

Active immunization: should be started immediately after passive immunization.

The main vaccine in use is:

Human diploid cell vaccine (HDCV)—now the vaccine of choice but, unfortunately, its cost limits its use to developed countries, which are not the countries that have the major problem of human rabies.

Contains: inactivated virus.

Prepared: in WI 38 or MRC-5 diploid human embryo lung cells.

Administered: intramuscularly or subcutaneously into the deltoid area of the upper arm in 6 doses spaced at 0, 3, 7, 14, 30 and 90 days.

Protection: effective; produces high levels of neutralizing antibody.

Safety: good: does not cause neuroparalytic complications—but there may be local reaction in around 15% of vaccinees.

Semple vaccine—the successor to the original Pasteur vaccine and still in use in many developing countries despite the risk of severe side-effects (see below).

Contains: virus inactivated by phenol.

Prepared: from infected brain tissue from rabbits, sheep or goats.

Administered: subcutaneously in 21 daily injections with later booster doses.

Protection: apparently effective.

Safety: severe neuroparalytic accidents due to allergic encephalomyelitis sometimes follow immunization due to the repeated injections of nervous tissue.

Suckling mouse brain vaccine is used in Latin America: it has shown a lower incidence of neurological side-effects.

Dog vaccines: inactivated virus vaccines (live attenuated vaccines are now rarely used).

Used: for immunization of dogs but cats and cattle in endemic areas—and occasionally other animals, for example, those in zoos, or particularly valuable stock, should be vaccinated.

Wild animals: trials of live attenuated virus distributed in bait have shown success in halting the spread of rabies in wildlife; this might in time lead to the eradication of the disease.

Pre-exposure vaccination

Veterinary surgeons, animal handlers, laboratory workers or others at high risk from rabies should be given two doses of diploid cell vaccine one month apart with a booster dose one year later; two booster doses should be given if they are exposed to infection.

Rabies antibody levels should be checked 3–4 weeks after the primary course.

MARBURG AND EBOLA VIRUS DISEASES

Marburg is an exceptionally severe disease which appeared in 1967 as a single outbreak initially involving laboratory workers in Marburg, Frankfurt and Belgrade. The patients had handled the tissues from the same batch of African green monkeys. Later, there were other cases in contacts of the patients. The monkeys were almost certainly infected during transit. Ebola—an equally severe disease—appeared amongst the populations of Sudan and Northern Zaire in 1976.

Clinical features

Clinically, both diseases are very severe, febrile illnesses with headaches, myalgia, a maculo-papular rash and haemorrhagic manifestations; other features are vomiting, diarrhoea, hepatitis, pharyngitis and signs of renal and CNS involvement. There is leucopenia and atypical lymphocytes and plasma cells in the blood. Disseminated intravascular coagulation was a feature of the Ebola cases.

The case fatality rate is high—considerably more than 50% in the Ebola outbreaks.

Infectiousness: a feature of both diseases is ability to spread directly from case to case: several of the infections have been in medical attendants of patients with the disease.

Epidemiology

Marburg disease appeared again in 1975 in two young people in South Africa. In 1976 there were severe outbreaks of a similar disease with many deaths in Sudan and Zaire. These outbreaks were due to a morphologically similar but antigenically different virus now named Ebola virus (after the river in the epidemic area in Zaire). The reservoir of Ebola virus now appears to be monkeys imported from the Phillipines to the USA in 1989–90.

Virology

1. Filoviruses
2. RNA viruses
3. Unusual virus particles, long, filamentous, with the ends bent or branching. Variable length, diameter 80 nm. Particles have surface spikes.
4. Grow in various tissue cultures without CPE but with intra-cytoplasmic inclusions
5. Pathogenic for guinea-pigs, monkeys and other laboratory animals.

Diagnosis

In the outbreaks, the diseases had a characteristic clinical picture. Confirmation of the virus aetiology in the original outbreak was obtained by isolating the virus in laboratory animals.

Isolation

Specimen: blood

Inoculate: guinea pigs (intraperitoneally) or cell cultures

Observe:
1. *guinea-pigs* for signs of febrile illness with detection of virus antigen by immunofluorescence in lesions in liver, lymph nodes or spleen
2. *cell cultures* for intracytoplasmic inclusions and by immunofluorescence.

Serology: complement fixation test.

ARENAVIRUSES

There are four human pathogenic arenaviruses:

1. Lymphocytic choriomeningitis
2. Lassa fever virus
3. Junin virus
4. Machupo virus.

The natural hosts of all four viruses are mice or rats. Infection is acquired by inhalation or ingestion of materials contaminated with rodent excreta. But Lassa fever can also be acquired by direct contact with a case of the disease.

LYMPHOCYTIC CHORIOMENINGITIS

The virus causes widespread natural infection in mice and is excreted in the urine and faeces of infected mice; transmission to man appears to be a rare event. The disease has also been acquired from pet and laboratory hamsters.

The disease is of interest from an immunological point of view since mice are not uncommonly infected in utero; when this happens they have a generalized infection with high titres of virus in all tissues and organs; however the mice remain symptomless although they later succumb to glomerulonephritis due to immune complex deposition in the kidney.

Clinical features

The most important syndrome in man is aseptic meningitis; sometimes meningo-encephalitis is seen; the virus also causes an influenza-like febrile illness.

LASSA FEVER

A serious febrile disease endemic in West Africa which was first reported in Lassa in Nigeria. The virus is highly infectious and spreads readily by contact—including to medical and nursing personnel looking after patients. Rats are the reservoir of the virus.

Clinical features

The illness is severe with fever, vomiting, cough, weakness and malaise; sore throat with ulcers in the mouth and pharynx and cervical lymphadenopathy are characteristic features; abdominal pain, myalgia with diarrhoea and headache are common and the blood count shows leucopenia; the case fatality is high—around a third of patients in reported outbreaks have died.

Symptomless infection: is now realized to be common among the population in geographical areas in Nigeria where the infection is present in wild rats, many of which have antibodies in their sera.

ARGENTINIAN AND BOLIVIAN HAEMORRHAGIC FEVERS

Due to Junin and Machupo viruses respectively. Clinically both are severe diseases with haemorrhagic, renal, cardiovascular and sometimes neurological symptoms. The reservoirs of both viruses are mouse-like rodents.The Argentinian disease is rural and spreads mainly during the maize harvest, from mice which inhabit the maize fields. The Bolivian disease is mostly acquired in houses.

Virology

1. Arenas are a large family of viruses
2. RNA viruses—the genome consists of two unique (i.e. not identical) virus-specific RNA segments
3. Medium-sized, 110 nm enveloped particles with internal granules which are host cell ribosomes
4. Grow in cell culture
5. Pathogenic for mice and guinea-pigs.

Diagnosis

Serology: complement fixation test (lymphocytic choriomeningitis). Immunofluorescence (Lassa fever).

Isolation

Specimens: blood, throat swabs, CSF etc.

Inoculate:

1. (for lymphocytic choriomeningitis) mice intracerebrally: observe for spasm of hind legs, tremors, convulsions and death
2. (for Lassa fever) Vero cell cultures: observe for CPE—or possibly virus antigen by immunofluorescence.

Vaccine

An attenuated Junin vaccine is under development.

HAEMORRHAGIC FEVER WITH RENAL SYNDROME (HFRS)

Originally called Korean haemorrhagic fever and first described in US soldiers in the Korean war. Now seen in two epidemic forms:

1. *Far East*: severe febrile illness with haemorrhage
2. *Scandinavia and Eastern Europe*: milder haemorrhagic fever with renal involvement; known as nephropathia epidemica.

Cause: Hantaan virus—a bunyavirus.

Epidemiology

A natural infection of mice—probably worldwide. Although mostly reported in epidemic form as described above, there have been occasional infections in other countries—including Britain. Some cases in Belgium were traced to infection in laboratory mice.

Diagnosis

Serology by immunofluorescence.

11 Herpesvirus diseases

There are a large number of herpesviruses. Most animal species, including man, are hosts for a particular herpesvirus and sometimes two or more viruses. All are morphologically identical and have the important property of remaining *latent*, in potentially viable form, within the cells of the host after primary infection. Latent virus persists for long periods of time—probably throughout life: some herpesviruses reactivate from time to time from the latent state to produce recurrent infection.

There are six recognized human herpesviruses:

1. Herpes simplex virus type 1
2. Herpes simplex virus type 2
3. Varicella-zoster virus
4. Cytomegalovirus
5. Epstein-Barr virus
6. Human herpes virus 6.

HERPES SIMPLEX VIRUS

Herpes simplex virus is unusual among viruses in causing a wide variety of clinical syndromes: the basic lesions are vesicles but these can take many different forms.

There are two types of herpes simplex virus—type 1 and type 2. The two viruses are biologically and serologically related but can be differentiated.

Type 1: the commonest, causes oro-facial lesions ('above the waist') but also a proportion of cases of genital herpes.

Type 2: the main cause of genital herpes.

Clinical features

Diseases due to the virus are in two categories:

1. *Primary*: when the virus is first encountered.
2. *Reactivation*: recurrent infections due to reactivation of latent virus.

Primary infections

Virtually everyone becomes infected with the virus but most primary infections are symptomless. Below are listed the main clinical manifestations when primary infection is accompanied by symptoms.

1. *Gingivo-stomatitis*: vesicles inside the mouth on the buccal mucosa and on the gums: these ulcerate and become coated with a greyish slough (Plate 3). Although this is the commonest primary disease, because kissing is the main route of virus spread, vesicles may be produced at other sites, most often on the head or neck.

2. *Herpetic whitlow*: due to implantation of the virus into the fingers: the lesion produced is very similar to a staphylococcal whitlow but the exudate is serous rather than purulent: an occupational hazard of doctors and nurses especially of anaesthetists or neurosurgical nurses, who deal with unconscious patients who are intubated: infection is acquired through contamination of the hands by virus in saliva or respiratory secretions.

3. *Conjunctivitis and keratitis*: primary herpes can involve the eye—both conjunctiva and cornea: the eyelids are generally swollen and there are often vesicles and ulcers on them.

4. *Kaposi's varicelliform eruption* is a superinfection of eczematous skin: mainly seen in young children, and sometimes a serious disease with a significant fatality rate.

5. *Acute necrotizing encephalitis*: herpes encephalitis is a very rare but extremely severe disease: clinically, it presents with the sudden onset of fever, mental confusion and headache: the main site of infection is the temporal lobe where the disease causes necrosis. Recently a milder form of herpes encephalitis with a better prognosis has been described—usually in children. It is uncertain if herpes encephalitis is a primary infection or a reactivation.

6. *Genital herpes*: a vesicular eruption of the genital area most often due to herpes simplex virus type 2: genital herpes is usually sexually transmitted. But note, genital herpes is due to type 1 virus in from a quarter to a third of cases.

7. *Neonatal infection*: severe generalized infection in neonates is usually acquired from a primary genital infection in the mother when no maternal antibody is present for the protection of the child: affected infants have jaundice, hepatosplenomegaly, thrombocytopenia and large vesicular lesions on the skin: there is a high case fatality rate: usually due to herpes simplex virus type 2 (unless acquired from a nurse or other person in the maternity ward who is suffering from a type 1 lesion).

8. *Generalized infection* in adults is a rare manifestation of primary infection with type 1 virus with disseminated vesicular skin lesions and virus in viscera and other body organs and tissues: *herpes hepatitis* has also been described.

Latency

During primary infection, the virus travels from the site of infection in the mouth to the trigeminal—and probably other cranial and cervical ganglia also. The mode of travel is via the nerves. Virus remains in the ganglia in a potentially viable state and in a proportion of people, *reactivates* to cause recurrent infection. Even in the absence of recurrent infection, virus can be isolated from the trigeminal ganglia in most people. The state of the virus in the ganglion neurones is in the form of virus DNA integrated into the cellular chromosomes. In genital herpes, type 2 becomes latent in the sacral ganglia.

Reactivation of virus is provoked by various stimuli including common colds, sunlight (possibly a result of exposure to ultraviolet light), pneumonia, stress, menstruation, etc. Reactivation recurs sporadically, sometimes often, throughout life.

Neutralizing antibody is formed after primary infection but does not prevent reactivation: virus is protected from serum antibody as it travels within the axons of sensory nerves to the site of recurrent infection. Reactivation does not stimulate a rise in titre of herpes antibody.

Clinical manifestations of reactivation:

1. *Cold sores*: vesicles round the mucocutaneous junctions of the nose and mouth are the most common: the vesicles progress to pustules with crust formation: the virus travels down the maxillary or mandibular branches of the trigeminal nerve to reach areas of the skin supplied by these nerves; herpetic vesicles can recur—but more rarely—at other sites on the skin: genital lesions also recur most often with type 2 virus—less often when the primary genital lesions are due to type 1 virus.

2. *Keratitis*: reactivation less commonly affects the eye: recurrent lesions are—at least at first—restricted to the cornea: virus reaches the cornea via the ophthalmic branch of the trigeminal nerve: lesions take the form of a branching or dendritic ulcer: if recurrence is frequent, scarring develops and in a few cases the disease progresses to a severe, destructive uveitis.

3. *Immunosuppressive therapy*: especially in patients with organ transplants is sometimes associated with severe, extensive cold sores; usually in the mouth, these may be necrotic and spread onto the face and into the oesophagus.

Epidemiology

Infection: is virtually universal in human populations and in elderly people the prevalence of antibody (indicating previous infection) is almost 100%. Although infection is widespread, herpes simplex is not seen in outbreaks.

Spread: by close personal contact, e.g. kissing (type 1 virus), sexual intercourse (type 2 virus).

Sources: generally people with herpetic lesions; however, carriers of latent virus from time to time secrete virus in their saliva without any symptoms and this may act as a source of (undetected) infection.

Age: Infection is most common in childhood and is usually symptomless: there is another peak in incidence during adolescence due to kissing as contact with the opposite sex increases.

Virology

1. Classified as an alphaherpesvirus

2. Roughly spherical particle with cubic symmetry, medium size—100 nm, with 162 projecting hollow-cored capsomeres; many of the particles are surrounded by a loose envelope of material partially derived from the host cell (Fig. 11.1)
3. Double-stranded DNA
4. Two types of virus (type 1s and 2) which share antigens in common (group-specific) but possess type-specific antigens also: although their DNA shows some homology, the two types of DNA can be readily distinguished by restriction enzyme analysis. Virus-specified proteins of the two viruses are produced in approximately equal numbers but can be distinguished by differences in their molecular weights when separated by electrophoresis in polyacrylamide gels
5. Grows in various tissue cultures with characteristic CPE with ballooning and rounding of cells
6. Grows on chorio-allantoic membrane with production of tiny white pocks
7. Pathogenic in laboratory animals, causing encephalitis.

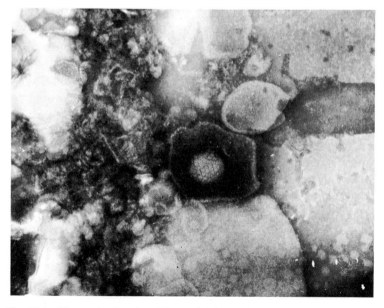

Fig. 11.1 Herpes simplex virus. The particle has cubic symmetry and the capsid is composed of hollow-cored capsomeres. There is a loose, baggy envelope. × 108 000. (Photograph by Dr E. A. C. Follett.)

Diagnosis

Isolation

Specimens: vesicle fluid, skin swab, saliva, conjunctival fluid, corneal scrapings, brain biopsy.

Inoculate: cell cultures, e.g. BHK21 (a hamster kidney cell line), human embryo lung cells.

Observe: for CPE of rounded cells.

Type: by neutralization test with standard antiserum or by immunofluorescence.

Serology

Complement fixation test: useful for diagnosing primary infections; difficult to interpret in recurrent infections because of high levels of existing antibody and because recurrences do not usually cause a rise in titre.

Direct demonstration: of virus or virus antigen in vesicle or other fluids or tissues by electron microscopy or immunofluorescence.

Treatment: (see also Ch.15)

Acyclovir: treatment of herpes simplex has been revolutionized by the introduction of this non-toxic drug which has a specific inhibitory action on herpes simplex virus replication.

Administered: intravenously, orally or topically

Indications: herpes encephalitis, severe or generalized herpes (given systemically); genital herpes (systemically or orally); dendritic ulcers, cold sores, possibly genital herpes topically; prophylaxis in immunocompromised patients.

Idoxuridine (0.1% solution): still used topically in the treatment of herpes keratitis.

VARICELLA-ZOSTER VIRUS

Varicella (chickenpox) and zoster (shingles—but also sometimes called 'herpes zoster') are different diseases due to the same virus.

Varicella is the *primary* illness.

Zoster is a *reactivation* of infection.

VARICELLA

Clinical features

Varicella—one of the common childhood fevers. A mild febrile illness with a characteristic vesicular rash; vesicles appear in successive waves so that lesions of different age are present together; the vesicles (in which there are giant cells) develop into pustules.

Complications are rare: post-infectious encephalomyelitis, haemorrhagic (fulminating) varicella; in adults, pneumonia is a relatively common and serious complication and may be followed by permanent pulmonary calcification.

Congenital varicella: exceedingly rare: maternal varicella in early pregnancy is occasionally followed, in the infant, by a syndrome of limb hypoplasia, muscular atrophy and cerebral and psychomotor retardation.

Perinatal or neonatal varicella: maternal varicella near the time of delivery may also affect the child: if the mother contracts varicella more than 5 days before delivery, the disease in the child is usually mild: this is because the child's disease is modified by placentally-transmitted early maternal antibody: when maternal varicella is contracted within 5 days of delivery, there is not time for maternal antibody to be produced and cross the placenta, and the child is liable to develop severe disease. Varicella may also be an unusually severe disease, with pneumonia, in pregnant women.

Immunity: attack is followed by solid and long lasting immunity to varicella—but *not to zoster*.

Epidemiology

Seasonal distribution: highest incidence is in late winter and early spring.

Spread: via nose and mouth by droplet infection from infectious saliva; virus is also present in skin lesions.

Varicella (cf. zoster) is an epidemic contagious disease; it may be acquired by contact with cases either of varicella or (less commonly) of zoster.

Zoster

A *reactivation* of virus latent in dorsal root or cranial nerve ganglia following—and usually many years after—childhood varicella. Virus travels down sensory nerves to produce painful vesicles in the area of skin (dermatome) enervated from the affected ganglion.

Virus: is present in the skin vesicles and in the ganglia involved (where there are cytopathic changes of cell destruction and marked inflammatory infiltration).

Adults: are affected much more often than children.

Ganglia: dorsal root ganglia—and therefore the thoracic nerves supplying the chest wall—are most often affected: there is a segmental rash which extends from the middle of the back in a horizontal strip round the side of the chest wall—'a belt of roses from hell'. (Plate 4).

Cranial zoster: when the ophthalmic nerve of the trigeminal ganglion is affected the rash is distributed within the skin supplied by that nerve, depending on the roots affected. This may cause a sharply demarcated area of lesions down one side of the forehead and scalp: in about half the patients, there are lesions in the eye.

Ramsay Hunt syndrome is a rare form of zoster: the eruption is on the tympanic membrane and the external auditory canal and there is often a facial nerve palsy.

Residual neuralgia—which may be severe—often follows zoster in the elderly.

Neurological signs are sometimes seen, e.g. paralysis.

Epidemiology

Zoster—unlike varicella—is not acquired by contact with cases of either varicella or zoster—although it may give rise to varicella in susceptible contacts.

Cases are *sporadic*: there is no seasonal distribution.

Virology

1. Classified as an alphaherpesvirus—one serological type
2. In the electron microscope the particle is that of a typical herpesvirus and is morphologically identical to that of herpes simplex
3. Double-stranded DNA virus
4. Grows slowly in tissue cultures of human cells (e.g. human embryo lung) with focal CPE.

Diagnosis

Serology: complement fixation test useful for both varicella (although laboratory diagnosis is rarely required because the clinical picture is so characteristic) and zoster: unlike reactivations of herpes simplex, zoster usually causes a rise in antibody titre.

Direct demonstration of typical herpesvirus particles in vesicle fluid by electron microscopy is a quick method of confirming a clinical diagnosis (but note, this does not distinguish varicella-zoster from herpes simplex virus).

Isolation: not routinely attempted: the virus is slow-growing, markedly cell-associated and difficult to passage: the CPE produced is focal and, with practice, easy to recognize. Immuno-fluorescence can be used to confirm the identity of the virus.

Treatment

Severe varicella or zoster (e.g. in the immunocompromised) responds well to acyclovir: the virus is less sensitive than herpes simplex but low toxicity means that dosage can be increased to produce inhibitory levels of the drug in blood and tissues.

CYTOMEGALOVIRUS

Cytomegalovirus rarely causes disease unless precipitating factors are present which lower the normal resistance of the host. Like rubella, cytomegalovirus can infect the fetus during maternal infection in pregnancy.

Symptomless infections are common: about 50% of the adult population has antibody to the virus almost always without developing any symptoms of disease.

Latency: the virus is known to reactivate from the latent state probably in polymorphonuclear leucocytes or lymphocytes but perhaps in other organs and cell types also.

There are two types of disease due to cytomegalovirus:

1. Congenital

A more difficult problem than congenital rubella because:

1. Maternal infection is almost always symptomless
2. The fetus can be damaged by infection in any of the three trimesters of pregnancy
3. Fetal infection can follow reactivation as well as primary maternal infection
4. Approximately 0.4% of British children are congenitally infected but most do not suffer sequelae (termination therefore presents ethical problems).

Clinical features

The majority of congenitally infected neonates show no signs or symptoms and diagnosis is made by virological tests. Many of the children develop normally but some show neurological sequelae later in life, principally:

1. deafness
2. mental retardation.

About a fifth of infected children do show clinical signs of infection and in some cases this take the form of the severe generalized—or cytomegalic inclusion—disease.

Severe generalized infection (cytomegalic inclusion disease)

Signs and symptoms: affected infants have jaundice, hepatosplenomegaly, blood dyscrasias such as thrombocytopenia and haemolytic anaemia; the brain is almost always involved and some infants have microcephaly: motor disorders are common; surviving infants are usually deaf and mentally retarded. Cytomegalovirus is probably the cause of about 10% of cases of microcephaly.

Affected organs: show characteristically enlarged cells (hence the prefix 'cytomegalo') with large intranuclear 'owl's eye' inclusions. Although this form of congenital cytomegalovirus infection is relatively rare, the effects are so severe that the disease represents a considerable medical and social problem.

2. Postnatal

Hepatitis

In young children, cytomegalovirus causes hepatitis with enlargement of the liver and disturbance of liver function tests; jaundice may or may not be present.

Infectious mononucleosis

In adults and in older children, infection may take the form of an illness—like infectious mononucleosis (see below) but with a negative Paul-Bunnell reaction and no lymphadenopathy or pharyngitis. There is fever, hepatitis and lymphocytosis with atypical lymphocytes in the peripheral blood; the syndrome is sometimes seen after transfusion with fresh unfrozen blood or platelets—presumably cytomegalovirus, which is occasionally present in the donor's blood, survives whereas it is normally inactivated by storage at 4°C.

Infection in the immunocompromised

Disseminated infection is sometimes seen when immunosuppressive therapy or severe debilitating disease, such as neoplasm is present to inhibit the normal immune response. There are usually widespread lesions involving lungs as well as other organs and tissues, e.g. adrenals, liver and alimentary tract. This is a major complication of transplantation surgery:

Renal transplant patients are subject to frequent infections with cytomegalovirus. Some of these are reactivations but recent evidence suggests that most are due to infection acquired from the donor organ. Many are not associated with signs or symptoms of disease. *Pneumonia*, and rarely, *retinitis* due to cytomegalovirus have, however, been reported in transplant patients.

Bone marrow transplant patients are even more susceptible to cytomegalovirus than those with renal grafts (possibly due to the greater immunosuppression with the former patients). Cytomegalovirus pneumonia is an important cause of death in them.

Virology

1. Classified as a betaherpesvirus
2. Electron microscopy—a typical herpesvirus particle
3. Double-stranded DNA
4. Grows slowly in cultures of human embryo lung cells with characteristic focal CPE and intranuclear 'owl's eye' inclusions.

Diagnosis

Isolation

Specimens: urine, throat swab.

Inoculate: human embryo lung cell cultures.

Observe: for characteristic CPE of foci of swollen cells; this may take from 2 to 3 weeks to appear.

Serology: immunofluorescence; ELISA tests for IgM; complement fixation test.

Demonstration: of typical intranuclear 'owl's eye' inclusions in cells of urinary sediment or other tissues.

Treatment

(i) Ganciclovir
(ii) Foscarnet.

Both are being used for severe cytomegalovirus infection but their efficacy is still uncertain. There is a high incidence of neutropenia associated with the use of ganciclovir.

EPSTEIN-BARR (EB) VIRUS

Epstein-Barr virus is named after the virologists who first observed it when examining cultures of lymphoblasts from Burkitt's lymphoma in the electron microscope. Recently, a variant of EB virus—type B—which differs from the original virus in its nuclear antigen has been described.

EB virus infection is widespread in human populations and most people have antibody to it by the time they reach adulthood. Type B virus, originally described in Africa and New Guinea, has recently been found in rural people in the USA.

Most infections are symptomless: especially if acquired during childhood; if infection is delayed until adult life there is greater likelihood of disease; this takes the form of *infectious mononucleosis* or glandular fever.

Persistence of virus: EB virus persists in latent form within lymphocytes following primary infection: the virus is present in the form of viral DNA—both free in the cytoplasm and integrated into the cellular chromosome. EB virus has oncogenic properties and transforms cells in vitro.

Human cancer: EB virus has a strong association, and is almost certainly a co-factor in causing Burkitt's lymphoma and nasopharyngeal carcinoma (see below).

INFECTIOUS MONONUCLEOSIS (glandular fever)

Clinical features

Incubation period: is long—from 4 to 7 weeks.

Route of infection: close or intimate contact, e.g. kissing; the virus has been demonstrated in cells in salivary secretions. The disease is most prevalent among young adults, especially student populations (of whom a sizeable minority have no antibody).

Signs and symptoms: low-grade fever with generalized lymphadenopathy and sore throat due to exudative tonsillitis; malaise, anorexia and tiredness to a severe degree are characteristic features; splenomegaly is common and most cases have abnormal liver function tests; a proportion have palpable enlargement of the liver and frank jaundice is not uncommon.

Mononucleosis: or—more correctly—a relative and absolute lymphocytosis is a diagnostic feature; at least 10% (and usually more) of the lymphocytes are atypical with enlarged misshapen nuclei and more cytoplasm than normal; the atypical lymphocytes are both B and T cells but mainly suppressor T-cells stimulated in a cytotoxic response against EB virus-infected B cells.

Paul-Bunnell test: infectious mononucleosis is characteristically associated with the appearance in the blood of heterophil antibodies to sheep erythrocytes; this antibody can be removed by absorption with ox erythrocytes but not with absorption with guinea-pig kidney. The differential absorption and the haemagglutination test with sheep erythrocytes constitute the Paul-Bunnell test which is diagnostic of infectious mononucleosis: development of other non-specific antibodies (e.g. rheumatoid factor and anti-i cold agglutinin) are also features of the disease.

EB virus antibody: is produced during infection but antibody is usually present before symptoms develop; the detection of EB virus-specific IgM is a useful confirmatory diagnostic test.

Duration: in most cases of infectious mononucleosis symptoms last from 2 to 3 weeks but, in a proportion, the illness may persist for weeks or even months.

EB virus infection in the immunocompromised: can cause severe lympho-proliferative disease which may be fatal and is characterized by infiltration of organs and tissues by immature B lymphocytes.

Purtillo's syndrome: fatal infectious mononucleosis with malignant lymphoma due to EB virus has been described in boys who suffer from this rare, congenital X-linked lympho-proliferative syndrome and who are immunodeficient.

EB virus and Burkitt's lymphoma

A highly malignant tumour which is common in African children. Primarily a tumour of lymphoid tissue but the earliest manifestations are often large tumours of the jaw and, in girls, sometimes of the ovaries; it spreads rapidly with widespread metastases.

There is a striking *geographical distribution*: the tumour is virtually confined to areas in Africa with holo-endemic malaria and in which disease-carrying mosquito vectors are found. Outside Africa, e.g. Western Europe and the USA, reported cases are sporadic and rare.

EB virus is certainly associated with Burkitt's lymphoma; the virus is found in cell cultures established from Burkitt's lymphoma and EB virus DNA is present—although not integrated—in the lymphoblasts of the tumour. Patients with Burkitt's lymphoma uniformly have antibody to the virus but so do a high proportion of normal people in any part of the world. Infection with EB virus is not, therefore, the sole cause of Burkitt's lymphoma.

The geographical distribution is perhaps explained by the fact that the areas where Burkitt's lymphoma is found are also areas in which the population is heavily infected with malaria. The effect of the parasites on the reticulo-endothelial system could cause an abnormal response to infection with EB virus. Instead of producing a benign proliferation of lymphoid tissue (as in infectious mononucleosis) the virus may become frankly oncogenic to produce malignant transformation in lymphoid tissue (as in Burkitt's lymphoma).

Nasopharyngeal carcinoma is a tumour which shows a striking geographical and probably racial distribution. For example, it is particularly common among the Southern Chinese. Nasopharyngeal carcinoma is also associated with EB virus and virus DNA is regularly present in the malignant epithelial cells of the tumour.

Virology

1. Classified as a gammaherpesvirus: two serological types, A and B
2. Electron microscopy—a typical herpesvirus particle. The capsid is antigenic—the viral capsid antigen—and is the basis for the main specific viral antibody test used in diagnosis
3. Double-stranded DNA virus
4. Grows in suspension cultures of human lymphoblasts
5. EB virus can be detected or isolated by its ability to 'transform' human lymphocytes into a continuously dividing line of cells. Transformed cells—including Burkitt's lymphoma cells (see above)—express EBNA (a virus nuclear antigen complex).

Diagnosis

Serology

1. Paul-Bunnell test
2. Demonstration of EB virus-specific IgM by immuno-fluorescence; the antibody tested is that directed against the viral capsid antigen.

Haematology: demonstration of atypical lymphocytes in the peripheral blood.

HUMAN HERPES VIRUS 6

Recently discovered, this virus (HHV-6) was found as a latent infection of lymphoid tissue. Infection is widespread, since there is a high incidence of antibody in normal populations, and is apparently acquired in early life.

Pathogenicity: still unclear: most infections appear to be symptomless.

 (i) *Exanthema subitum* (also known as *roseola infantum*): this mild facial rash in small babies seems to be associated with HHV-6 infection
(ii) *Mononucleosis with cervical lymphadenopathy*: has been described in a few adults undergoing primary infection.

12 Childhood fevers

Mumps, measles, rubella

Mumps, measles and rubella are, with varicella, the common childhood fevers. Measles has been, at least partially, controlled by vaccination and this has altered its traditional epidemiology. Until 1988, rubella vaccination was aimed at protecting girls in their teens against the risk of fetal infection while not interfering with naturally-acquired immunity. A most significant advance is the recent introduction of a combined, live, attenuated measles, mumps and rubella (MMR) vaccine.

More recently, another childhood fever, erythema infectiosum, due to a human parvovirus has been recognized.

MUMPS

Clinical features

Incubation period: relatively long—18 to 21 days.

Clinically: classical mumps is a febrile illness with inflammation of salivary glands causing characteristic swelling of parotid and submaxillary glands.

Aseptic meningitis: (less often meningoencephalitis) is a frequent neurological complication of mumps; occasionally there is muscular weakness or paralysis. Mumps meningitis is not accompanied by parotitis in 50% of cases. *Nerve deafness* is a rare complication.

Other complications: *orchitis*, *pancreatitis* and—rarely—*oophoritis* and *thyroiditis* are seen in association with mumps; about 20% of adult males who contract mumps develop orchitis.

Immunity: an attack is followed with solid and long-lasting immunity; second attacks are very rare.

Mumps is a generalized infection by a virus with a predilection for the CNS (neurotropism) and for glandular tissue.

Epidemiology

Spread is by droplet infection with infectious respiratory secretions.

Seasonal prevalence: highest in winter and spring.

Age distribution: more frequent in children aged from 5 to 15 years but not uncommon in young adults: outbreaks have been reported in recruit populations.

Infectiousness: lower then measles; as a result infection in childhood is not as common as measles and a significant proportion of adults are non-immune.

Adults: tend to have more severe disease and orchitis and oophoritis are considerably more common after puberty.

Epidemics of mumps were seen every 3 years followed by years when the prevalence of infection was low. The introduction of MMR vaccine can be expected to have a dramatic effect on the prevalence of mumps in the future.

Virology

1. Paramyxovirus, one serological type
2. RNA virus—single-stranded, negative sense RNA
3. Enveloped particles, rather large in size—110 to 170 nm; helical symmetry
4. Haemagglutinates fowl erythrocytes
5. Grows in amniotic cavity of chick embryo and in monkey kidney and other tissue cultures with haemadsorption.

Diagnosis

Serology (widely used):

Complement fixation test: Two antigens are used:

1. 'S' or soluble antigen (the nucleoprotein core of the virus particle)
2. 'V' or viral antigen (found on the surface of the virus particle).

Antibody to 'S' antigen tends to diminish sooner than antibody to 'V' antigen; it can therefore be a useful indicator of recent infection. 'V' antibody usually persists for years.

Isolation (mainly used for diagnosis of mumps meningitis).

Specimens: CSF, possibly throat washings.

Inoculate: monkey kidney tissue cultures.

Observe: for haemadsorption of fowl erythrocytes.

Identify virus: by inhibition of haemadsorption or haemagglutination with standard antiserum.

Vaccine: see MMR vaccine page 119

MEASLES

Clinical features

Measles is the most common of childhood fevers; in uncomplicated cases it is a mild disease but complications are relatively frequent.

Prodromal symptoms are respiratory, e.g. nasal discharge and suffusion of the eyes.

The main illness of measles follows; fever—which may be high—with a maculopapular rash lasting from two to five days: the rash is an enanthem (as well as an exanthem) and characteristic spots (Koplik's spots) appear in the buccal mucosa inside the cheek and mouth.

Immunity following measles is life-long: but note, measles itself has a suppressive effect on the immune system.

Complications

1. Respiratory
2. Neurological

1. **Respiratory infections**: are the most common and are seen in about 4% of patients; these include bronchitis, bronchiolitis, croup and bronchopneumonia; *otitis media* is also seen in about 2.5% of cases. Before the advent of antibiotics these

infections were more frequent and were largely responsible for the mortality associated with measles.

Giant cell pneumonia: a rare complication, seen in children immunodeficient or with chronic debilitating disease; due to direct invasion of the lungs by measles virus and usually fatal: there are numerous multinucleated giant cells in the lungs at post-mortem.

2. ***Neurological complications***: two types of encephalitis are seen:

(i) *Encephalitis or post-infectious encephalomyelitis*: a serious condition which follows measles in about one in every 1000 cases; the mortality rate is about 50% and many survivors have residual neurological symptoms. Encephalitis commonly presents with drowsiness, vomiting, headache and convulsions.

(ii) *Subacute sclerosing panencephalitis*: a rare but severe, chronic, neurological disease seen in children and young adults. The presenting symptoms are of personality and behavioural changes with intellectual impairment; the disease progresses to convulsions, myoclonic movements and increasing neurological deterioration leading to coma and death. Due to persistent infection with measles virus following primary and usually uncomplicated measles several years previously; affected children have high titres of measles antibody in their serum and both IgM and IgG measles-specific antibody in the CSF.

At post mortem, there are numerous intranuclear inclusions throughout the brain: measles virus has been grown from brain tissue.

Epidemiology

The attack rate in measles is high: in former years, before vaccination, virtually everybody in Britain under the age of 15 years had had the disease. When the disease has been introduced into isolated communities where it was not endemic and the entire population was susceptible, attack rates of more than 99% have been recorded.

Spread is by inhalation of respiratory secretions from patients in the early stages of the disease.

Epidemics: measles in Britain used to appear in epidemics every second year—probably because in two years sufficient new susceptible hosts had been born into the community for the virus to become epidemic again; in non-epidemic years measles was endemic but the number of cases was lower than in the epidemic years.

The introduction of measles vaccine caused a marked reduction in the prevalence both of measles and measles encephalitis.

In countries like Britain, where there is little poverty and malnutrition, measles is a mild disease with a low mortality rate.

In under-developed countries, e.g. West Africa, measles remains a severe disease and a major cause of death in childhood.

Virology

1. Paramyxovirus, one serological type
2. RNA virus—single-stranded, negative sense RNA
3. Enveloped particles, rather large, 120 to 250 nm; helical symmetry
4. Haemagglutinates and haemolyses monkey erythrocytes
5. Grows in human embryo and primary monkey kidney cells with syncytial CPE of multinucleated giant cells.

Diagnosis

Serology: complement fixation test; detection of measles IgM by immunofluorescence; in subacute sclerosing panencephalitis, the diagnosis can be confirmed by demonstration of measles antibody in the CSF.

Direct demonstration of viral antigen by immunofluorescence in nasopharyngeal aspirates

Isolation

Specimens: throat washings, blood, urinary sediment, etc.

Culture: best are primary human embryo kidney cells.

Observe: for characteristic CPE.

Note: Laboratory confirmation is rarely necessary in measles as the clinical features are characteristic and easily recognized.

Vaccine: see MMR vaccine page 119

Normal immunoglobulin

Normal immunoglobulin is derived by pooled human sera and therefore contains measles antibody: it can be used to confer passive immunity to infants and other unusually susceptible individuals who have been in contact with cases of measles.

RUBELLA

Rubella is a mild childhood fever but if infection is contracted in early pregnancy the virus can cause severe congenital abnormalities and disease in the fetus.

Clinical features

A mild febrile illness with a macular rash which spreads down from the face and behind the ears; there is usually pharyngitis and enlargement of the cervical—and especially the posterior cervical—lymph glands.

Virus is present in both blood and pharyngeal secretions and is excreted during the incubation period for up to seven days before the appearance of the rash.

Infection is symptomless in a proportion of cases.

Complications are rare: post-infectious encephalomyelitis, thrombocytopenic purpura and arthralgia or painful joints.

Congenital infection

The teratogenic properties of the virus were first discovered in Australia in 1941: Gregg (an ophthalmologist) noticed an increased number of cases of congenital cataract following an epidemic of rubella: affected infants had been born to mothers with a history of rubella in early pregnancy and he concluded that early maternal rubella could cause congenital defects in the offspring.

Congenital defects follow rubella only in the first 16 weeks of pregnancy; after that rubella does not damage the fetus.

The main defects are a triad of:

Cataract
Nerve deafness
Cardiac abnormalities (e.g. patent ductus arteriosus, ventricular septal defect, pulmonary artery stenosis, Fallot's tetralogy).

However affected infants have various other disorders due to generalized infection which, together with the defects, are known as *the rubella syndrome* (Plate 5); these are:

Hepatosplenomegaly
Thrombocytopenic purpura
Low birth weight
Mental retardation
Jaundice
Anaemia
Lesions in the metaphyses of the long bones.

The incidence of defects after maternal rubella in the first three months of pregnancy has varied from 10% to 54% in different studies. Maternal rubella at this time also is associated with a higher proportion of abortions and stillbirths.

Time of infection: the severity and multiplicity of defects are increased when infection is in the earliest weeks of pregnancy.

The frequency of both deafness and defective vision further increases as congenitally-infected children grow up—probably due to easier recognition of these defects in older children.

Subacute sclerosing panencephalitis has been reported as a rare, late, complication of congenital rubella.

Infants with the rubella syndrome have IgM antibody to rubella virus and therefore are immunologically competent (the maternal antibody which crosses the placenta is IgG antibody).

Immunity after rubella. There is good immunity after naturally and vaccine-acquired rubella but it is not solid and reinfections are well documented. Although less of a risk to the fetus than primary infection, congenital infections have been reported as a result of maternal reinfection.

Epidemiology

Mainly attacks children under 15 years of age but a proportion of people reach adult life without being infected so that rubella in adults is not uncommon; before vaccination about 15% of women of child-bearing age had not been infected and were therefore non-immune.

Infection is endemic in the community with epidemics every few years: the most extensive outbreak recorded was in the USA in 1964 when there were 1 800 000 cases. But note, rubella has shown a very marked reduction in the USA due to the policy there of vaccinating both boys and girls.

Virology

1. A non-arthropod-borne togavirus, one serological type
2. RNA virus—single-stranded, negative sense RNA
3. Pleomorphic-enveloped particles, medium size—50 to 75 nm; helical symmetry
4. Haemagglutinates bird erythrocytes
5. Grows in a rabbit kidney cell line—RK 13 with production of CPE and in other tissue cultures but without CPE.

Diagnosis

Laboratory diagnosis is now widely used for confirmation of the diagnosis of rubella—usually in a pregnant woman or in suspected congenital rubella; also used to detect non-immune women who may be offered vaccination.

Serology

IgM antibody: recent infection with rubella virus is best diagnosed by the demonstration of IgM rubella antibody in a single sample of blood; detected by ELISA or by immuno-fluorescence.

Haemagglutination-inhibition test: quite a sensitive technique for detecting rubella antibody: active rubella (e.g. in pregnancy) can be diagnosed by demonstration of a rising titre of IgG. Specimens need only be 3 days apart.

Isolation: (most often used for the diagnosis of congenital rubella in the fetus.)

Inoculate: RK 13 (rabbit kidney) or SIRC (rabbit cornea) cell lines.

Observe: for CPE.

Single radial haemolysis: widely used for detecting immunity in pregnant women or in women at special risk e.g. children's nurses, schoolteachers: it does not measure antibody titre and is not suitable for the diagnosis of rubella.

MMR VACCINATION

*Combined measles, mumps and rubella vaccination i*s now recommended for all infants in the second year of life. This policy augments, but does not in the meantime replace, the present vaccination of adolescent schoolgirls and non-immune women of child-bearing age.

The MMR vaccination programme aims to eradicate measles, mumps and rubella viruses from Britain. A high uptake of vaccine will increase herd immunity to the level at which too few susceptible (i.e. non-immune) hosts remain to enable the circulation—and survival—of the three viruses in the community.

Rubella vaccine on its own will continue to provide protection to schoolgirls and to women of child-bearing age found to be non-immune.

MMR Vaccine

Indications: given to all children in the second year of life: also recommended at school-entry to 'speed up' the immunization of the children in the gap between the girls in the older 11–14 year schedule and the MMR-vaccinated babies.

Contains: live, attenuated virus strains:

1. Measles ⎫
2. Mumps ⎬ both prepared in chick embryo cell culture
3. Rubella—prepared in human diploid cell culture.

Administered: one dose, subcutaneously or intramuscularly.

Protection: apparently excellent: immunity seems to be long-lasting, but careful surveillance will be necessary to monitor that immunity persists over many years.

Reactions: generally mild: fever, malaise, rash, coryza (due to the measles virus component); sometimes with parotitis and arthralgia (associated with the mumps and rubella virus components respectively): febrile convulsions.

Rarely, meningo-encephalitis: due to mumps virus: associated with raised lymphocytes in the CSF (from which vaccine-type mumps virus can usually be isolated).

Contraindications:

(i) *Pregnancy*; in women, pregnancy must be avoided for one month after vaccination
(ii) *Immunodeficiency*: due to immunosuppressive therapy, disease (leukaemia, other malignant disease) or other causes
(iii) *Hypersensitivity* to eggs.

Rubella vaccine

Indications: girls aged 11–14 years: women of child-bearing age who are non-immune (e.g. detected by antenatal screening for rubella antibody).

Contains: live attenuated rubella virus.

Administered: one dose subcutaneously or intramuscularly.

Protection: good (but, note, occasional reports of infection in previously vaccinated women have been reported).

Reactions: rare, and generally mild—fever, rash, cervical lymphadenopathy: arthralgia—especially in adult women.

Contraindications:

Pregnancy; pregnancy must be avoided for one month after vaccination.

Passive immunization with rubella-specific immunoglobulin may have some attenuating or prophylactic effect in rubella. It may be considered for use in maternal rubella if termination is refused.

ERYTHEMA INFECTIOSUM

This disease (also called 'slapped cheek' or 'fifth disease') is due to human parvovirus, B19.

Clinical features

Signs and symptoms: fever, rash. The rash is erythematous, most intense on the cheeks were there is marked redness, hence the name 'slapped cheek disease', and circumoral pallor. The rash on the body and limbs may become maculopapular: lesions fade from the centre leaving the periphery red so that the rash develops with a characteristic reticular or lace-like pattern. There is a mild generalized lymphadenopathy and, especially in women, arthralgia with swelling and pain in the joints. The syndrome is, clinically, like rubella.

Aplastic crises: B19 virus has a predilection for the haemopoietic cells of the bone marrow causing aplastic crises. These have been mainly described in patients, most often children, with chronic haemolytic anaemias such as sickle cell anaemia, hereditary spherocytosis, thalassaemia. There is evidence that previously healthy people also show transient bone marrow 'arrest' during the course of infection.

Symptomless infection: appears to be common—probably around 20% of those infected have no symptoms.

Hydrops fetalis: like rubella, B19 virus can infect the fetus during the course of maternal infection. Many congenital infections are symptomless and the fetus develops normally. However, especially from the 10th to the 20th week of pregnancy, when the fetus seems most vulnerable, the virus can cause severe fetal infection and death with a catastrophic fall in the haemaglobin level. The affected fetus resembles the hydrops fetalis associated with a rhesus blood group incompatibility, so that the parvovirus syndrome is called *non-immune hydrops fetalis*.

Persistent B19 infection: causing chronic anaemia has been reported in children with acute lymphocytic leukaemia and other forms of immunodeficiency.

Epidemiology

Epidemics: outbreaks of infection are seen in the community approximately every 4 years. Between outbreaks, B19 virus is endemic causing sporadic infections.

Spread: probably by inhalation of infected respiratory secretions.

Seasonal prevalence: most common in late winter and early spring.

Age: the peak incidence of infection is in childhood during the early school years—from 5–10 years old.

Virology

1. Human parvovirus. B19 is one of the three serologically different human parvoviruses and the only one known to cause disease: classed in the genus of autonomously replicating parvoviruses
2. DNA virus. Single-stranded DNA. The virus genetic organization is interesting, because populations of virus show, in roughly equal measure, particles which contain either positive or negative sense DNA molecules respectively
3. Electron microscopy. Small featureless icosahedral particles 18–26 nm in diameter
4. Haemagglutinates
5. Does not grow in tissue culture cells: there are no susceptible laboratory animals.

Diagnosis

Serology: ELISA or RIA for virus-specific IgM.

Direct demonstration: in tissues, blood

   (i) *Virus particles* in tissues and blood by electron microscopy
   (ii) *Virus DNA*: by radioactive probe.

Note: The virus cannot be cultivated in vitro. The diagnostic tests listed above have been developed by molecular biotechnology.

13 Poxvirus diseases

Most, possibly all, animal species are hosts to their own pox-viruses. Man's was smallpox—one of the most fatal of all virus infections. Yet it was defeated—for three reasons:

1. Man was the only host animal
2. There was an effective vaccine against it (originally discovered by Jenner in 1796)
3. By the mid 20th century there were only a limited number of areas of endemic infection.

Eradication

In 1967 the World Health Organization embarked on a Smallpox Eradication campaign. This was based on a policy of 'search and containment', i.e. the isolation of cases and the tracing and vaccination of contacts. There was continuing and long-term surveillance of previously endemic areas before these were declared smallpox-free. The main endemic areas were India, Pakistan and Bangladesh and, in Africa, Ethiopia and Somalia. The campaign was outstandingly successful and smallpox has now been eradicated: the World Health Organization declared the world free from smallpox in May 1980.

OTHER POXVIRUS DISEASES

Molluscum contagiosum

A low grade infection in man characterized by reddish, waxy papules on the skin—most often seen in the axilla or on the trunk. It is a fairly common infection in children and is spread by close contact, e.g. at swimming baths; the lesions contain numerous poxvirus particles which can be seen in the electron microscope; the lesions resolve spontaneously in 4 to 6 weeks.

123

Orf or contagious pustular dermatitis

An infection of sheep and goats: occasionally transmitted to hands of animal workers causing chronic granulomatous lesions; diagnosed by characteristic oval particles in electron microscope with criss-cross surface banding.

Paravaccinia or pseudocowpox

The virus appears to be identical with orf virus; it causes lesions on udders of cows and is occasionally transmitted to hands of animal workers.

Monkeypox

This is a disease resembling mild smallpox which is due to a natural pox virus of monkeys; it is seen in Africa among people with frequent contact with monkeys.

Tanapox

This virus is probably also acquired from contact with monkeys and, in humans, produces scanty vesicular lesions on the skin which do not progress to pustules. Epidemics have been reported in East Africa.

Virology

1. Pox viruses include the human viruses smallpox (variola) and molluscum contagiosum, vaccinia (origin uncertain—probably originally derived from horsepox which died out as a natural infection in the 19th century) together with cowpox and other animal pox viruses
2. DNA viruses—double-stranded DNA
3. Large viruses, approximately 250 to 300 nm: two morphological types of particle:
   (i) Large, brick-shaped (vaccinia, molluscum contagiosum)
   (ii) Large, oval with criss-cross surface bonding (orf, paravaccinia)
4. Some grow in tissue cultures, others do not (e.g. molluscum contagiosum)
5. Many produce characteristic pocks or visible lesions on the chorio-allantoic membrane of the chick embryo.

14 Viral hepatitis

Hepatitis is a common complication of infection with many different viruses—for example, yellow fever, cytomegalovirus and Epstein-Barr virus infection, and congenital rubella. But a different group of viruses infect the liver as the primary target organ to cause the disease 'viral hepatitis'. Originally thought to be due to two viruses (hepatitis A and B), five hepatitis viruses are now recognized—and there may be more. These five are listed below:

Table 14.1 Hepatitis viruses

	A	B	C	D	E
Virus genome	SS RNA	DS DNA	SS RNA	SS RNA (defective: hepatitis B acts as helper)	Unknown
Transmission	faecal–oral food, water	sex, blood, congenital	blood, (other?)	as for hepatitis B	water-borne (often epidemic)

Hepatitis due to these viruses presents clinically in a similar fashion, and although the incubation period may be a differentiating feature, this is of little help in diagnosis unless the time of contracting the virus is known. Nowadays sensitive and reliable laboratory tests are available for the diagnosis of all these viruses, with the exception of hepatitis E.

Clinical features

Symptoms: the cardinal symptom is of jaundice which is often low grade. Marked anorexia, nausea and malaise precede the jaundice.

Jaundice: is obstructive in type with raised bilirubin, dark bile-containing urine and pale stools.

Transaminases: liver function tests are abnormal with raised transaminase levels—i.e. ALT (or alanine aminotransferase)—in the serum.

Duration: variable, but usually 2–3 weeks.

Anicteric hepatitis: is common in all forms of viral hepatitis: there is disturbance of liver function tests, fever, and the other constitutional signs and symptoms, but no frank jaundice.

Symptomless infection: is also common: a particular problem in control because virus is excreted by patients without recognition that they are infected.

Complications:

(i) *Massive liver necrosis* ('acute yellow atrophy') leading to liver failure, coma and, not infrequently, death. Seen with hepatitis A—although rarely—and, sometimes, hepatitis B.
(ii) *Chronic hepatitis*: a not uncommon complication following hepatitis B and hepatitis C (see below).

HEPATITIS A

Clinical features

Incubation period: long, about 4 weeks.

Age incidence: mainly children aged 5 to 15 years: but food-borne outbreaks may predominantly affect adults.

Clinically: generally a milder disease than hepatitis B: massive liver necrosis is a rare complication: overall case fatality rate in hepatitis A is 0.1%.

Alimentary infection: the site of entry and primary multiplication is the gut: virus then spreads to infect the liver where it multiplies in hepatocytes.

Virus is excreted in the faeces for about 2 weeks before the onset of jaundice, but for only a few days after the onset of symptoms.

Viraemia: blood is briefly infectious, but is an uncommon source of infection.

Antibody: appears at the time of onset of jaundice.

Epidemiology

World-wide in distribution: endemic in most countries and especially common in the tropics; more common in rural than urban communities. Epidemics appear from time to time, some of which are associated with sewage contamination of food or water.

Spread: there are two main routes of infection:

1. *Case-to-case spread* via the faecal–oral route, the most common route of the spread of the disease; symptomless excretors may be an important—because undetected—source of infection.
2. *Via contaminated food and water*: numerous outbreaks have been described due to contamination of food-stuffs by a food-handler who is excreting virus or due to pollution of water by infected sewage. *Raw shellfish* (especially oysters) which have become contaminated by growing in sewage-polluted water have been responsible for several large outbreaks.

Seasonal: infection is more common in autumn and winter.

Decline: the incidence of hepatitis A in Europe (especially in Britain) declined sharply in the decade of the 1970s, but increased again in the 1980s. The decrease in incidence was not observed in underdeveloped or tropical countries.

Virology

1. A picornavirus
2. RNA—single-stranded, positive sense RNA
3. Small spherical particles, 27 nm
4. Reported to be relatively heat-resistant, i.e. withstands 60°C for 30 minutes
5. Grows, but only very slowly and with difficulty, in tissue culture: there is no CPE
6. Infects chimpanzees and a few other primates, e.g. marmosets.

Diagnosis

Serology: detection of virus-specific IgM by RIA or ELISA.

Demonstration of virus in stools by electron microscopy.

Passive immunization

Normal immunoglobulin protects people exposed to hepatitis A; *there is no immunity for 2 weeks after inoculation,* but the immunity thereafter lasts for 4 to 6 months: recommended for anyone travelling to tropical countries where hepatitis A is endemic and common.

HEPATITIS B

Clinical features

Incubation period: is long—from 2 to 5 months.

Sex incidence: predominantly seen in males.

Onset: typically, rather insidious.

Clinical course: tends to be a more severe disease than hepatitis A.

Viraemia: virus and virus surface antigen (see below) are present in the blood during the acute phase—and, not uncommonly, persist for longer.

Epidemiology

Hepatitis B was a major cause of post-transfusion hepatitis in Britain, but is now rare as a result of screening blood donations. Blood may be highly infectious and one extensive epidemic of infection followed the use during the Second World War of yellow fever vaccine, which included human serum as a stabilizing agent. Infection can also be spread by the use of communal or inadequately sterilized syringes and needles.

Drug abusers: are at particular risk from hepatitis B; infection is transmitted by sharing of unsterilized syringes used for intravenous administration of drugs: infection is endemic in the drug-abusing community.

Sexual transmission: patients—especially male homosexuals—attending clinics for sexually-transmitted diseases show a higher incidence of antigen and antibody to the virus than the normal population and the disease itself is considerably more common in male homosexuals than in other groups in the community.

Tattooing and acupuncture: have also been the source of outbreaks of hepatitis B; less obviously, the disease was common amongst *track runners* in Sweden, apparently because of communal bathing or by direct inoculation resulting from scratches and minor abrasions caused by running through thickets.

Non-parenteral spread: some cases of hepatitis B, especially in young children, appear to be due to non-parenteral transmission —possibly through close personal contact.

Renal dialysis units: hepatitis B has in the past been a particular problem in renal units: infection is introduced by the blood transfusions required by the patients and spreads from them to other patients and staff. Hospital staff involved have been not only doctors and nurses but also biochemistry and haematology MLSOs who handle samples of infected blood. There have been several hospital-based outbreaks of infection, although most have been mild with no deaths: in others, like that in Edinburgh Royal Infirmary in which there was a 30% case fatality rate, the mortality has been high.

Carriers of hepatitis B virus: in Africa and Asia symptomless carriage is common—up to 15% of some populations: in Britain the prevalence of carriage is about 0.1%.

Animal hepatitis B counterparts: diseases similar to human hepatitis B exist in the animal world where some species of ducks, squirrels and woodchucks are natural hosts to viruses which resemble hepatitis B in their properties. Primary liver cell cancer is associated with infection in woodchucks and ducks.

Acute hepatitis B in pregnancy: can result in infection of the infant; the virus is transmitted transplacentally in utero or during delivery; the infected babies become chronic carriers of hepatitis B antigen in their blood and around half of them develop persistent hepatitis. Infection of the newborn infant is less common if the mother is a symptomless carrier of hepatitis B virus or antigen than if she has acute hepatitis B; however, more infants become infected in the months after birth presumably due to close contact with their infected mothers.

Sequelae

Attacks of hepatitis B are followed—in around 3% of cases—by the development of *chronic active hepatitis*; a proportion of patients with chronic active hepatitis have evidence of asymptomatic hepatitis B virus carriage. This severe disease is associated with liver dysfunction and a fluctuating course leading in many cases to cirrhosis and progressive liver failure. However, hepatitis B is not the only cause of chronic active hepatitis; in fact probably only a minority of cases of chronic active hepatitis are due to previous hepatitis B. The newly available test for hepatitis C has shown that this virus, too, can cause chronic active hepatitis.

Chronic persistent hepatitis is a benign and self-limiting disease which sometimes follows hepatitis B; there are mild inflammatory signs in the liver but symptoms are minor or absent; this disease too is probably associated with previous hepatitis B in a minority of patients—most cases being due to other, often unknown, causes.

Cancer

Hepatocellular carcinoma: or primary liver cell cancer is strongly associated with carriage of hepatitis B virus. The virus DNA has been shown to integrate into liver cell chromosomes (a prerequisite for oncogenicity). Hepatocellular cancer is rare in Europe but common in Africa and Asia and it is likely that, world-wide, hepatitis B virus is, therefore, a major cause of cancer. The animal counterparts of human hepatitis B virus, which cause tumours in the host species, are further evidence of the oncogenicity of this family of viruses.

Virology

1. Hepadnavirus
2. DNA virus—double-stranded DNA but with single-stranded regions
3. *Electron microscopy*: see Figure 14.1: roughly spherical particles (known as Dane particles) 42 nm in diameter. *Dane particles* are the virions of hepatitis B virus: they contain a particle-associated DNA polymerase: infected blood also shows 22 nm spherical particles—much more abundant than Dane particles —and tubular structures both of which are aggregates of virus coat protein.

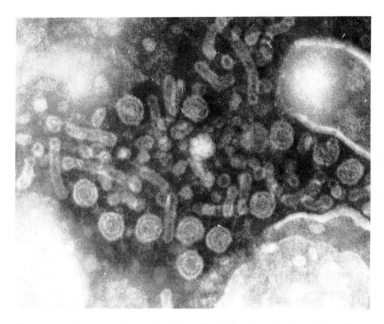

Fig. 14.1   Electron micrograph of hepatitis B virus showing large 42 nm Dane particles, smaller 22 nm spherical and tubular particles. × 220 000. (Photograph by Dr E. A. C. Follett.)

Antigenic structure

Hepatitis B virus has the following antigens:

HBsAg: the surface antigen found also on the 22 nm particles
HBcAg: the antigen of the inner core of the Dane particle
HBeAg: also part of the core of the Dane particle and strongly associated with infectivity (see below).

Antigenic subtypes: the 4 subtypes of hepatitis B antigen are based on HBsAg:

adw
adr
ayw
ayr

All share the group-specific determinant *a* in addition to the allelic *d* and *y* (never found together) and—although less often tested—allelic *w* and *r* (which are also mutually exclusive).

Subtype distribution: the predominant subtype of hepatitis B antigen in various situations is as follows:

Symptomless blood donors	*ad*
Acute hepatitis	*ad* and *ay*
Renal units	*ay*
Drug abusers	*ay*

HBe antigen: this antigen is usually present—although briefly—in patients' blood in the acute phase of hepatitis B; its presence in the blood of cases or carriers correlates with infectivity of the blood. But, note, absence of *e* antigen cannot guarantee that the blood concerned is non-infectious. The continuing presence of *e* antigen also correlates with chronic liver disease and it is found in the blood of a high proportion of patients with chronic active hepatitis following hepatitis B. Conversely: anti-*e* antibody is usually present in healthy carriers and the infectivity of blood containing it is low.

Antibody to hepatitis B core antigen (anti HBc) appears early in infection—and disappears earlier than *antibody to hepatitis B surface antigen* (anti HBs) which appears later during convalescence: antibody to hepatitis B surface antigen is present in about 2% of the British population. The incidence is higher in certain groups, i.e. haemophiliac patients, people with a past history of hepatitis B, homosexual men, drug abusers and certain groups of hospital staff.

Diagnosis

Serology

Detection of hepatitis B surface antigen (HBsAg) by RIA , ELISA test: less sensitive is reversed passive haemagglutination in which turkey erythrocytes are coated with hepatitis B antibody and the patient's serum is then tested for ability to agglutinate the cells.

Additional useful tests:

(i)   anti HBc (IgM) by ELISA—distinguishes active infection from long-term carriage in HBsAg-positive people

(ii) *e* antigen (HBeAg) by RIA or ELISA—a marker of infectiousness.

Tests of immunity (or previous infection): detection of anti HBs by RIA or ELISA.

Vaccine

Available for those at special risk (e.g. laboratory staff, haemophiliac patients, patients and staff in institutions for the mentally subnormal, renal units, babies born to carrier mothers etc.).

Contains: HBsAg, now prepared by genetic engineering (early vaccine was purified from the blood of carriers): adsorbed onto alum.

Administered: intramuscularly in three doses at intervals of one and then six months.

Protection: apparently good, but may not be long-lasting.

Safety: good.

Response to vaccine is not always satisfactory and it is wise to check antibody levels after completion of the course.

Babies: born to HBsAg-positive mothers should be immunized within a few hours of birth: vaccine should be given simultaneously, but at a different site, with hepatitis B specific immunoglobulin.

Passive immunization: injection of hepatitis B specific immunoglobulin gives partial but significant protection against the disease: it should be used in people exposed in a single episode involving a high risk of infection, e.g. accidental inoculation of blood suspected or known to contain hepatitis B virus: active immunization should be started as soon as possible.

HEPATITIS C

It has been known that blood transfusion was followed, in around 1% of cases, by hepatitis that was neither A nor B (non A-non B hepatitis). Only very recently has a test for antibody to this virus become available and, as yet, only to specialist laboratories.

Clinical features and epidemiology

Post transfusion hepatitis: generally a somewhat milder form of hepatitis than hepatitis B and with a shorter incubation period (usually 6 to 8 weeks).

Antibody to the virus (or at least that detected by the new test): develops late—up to 6 months after the onset of jaundice.

Blood donors: 0.5–1.0% in Britain have antibody to hepatitis C.

Haemophiliacs: the majority have evidence of past infection (i.e. presence of antiviral antibody) indicating frequent contamination of factor VIII concentrate.

Drug-abusers: usually have a high prevalence of antibody indicating frequent exposure to infection.

Hepatocellular carcinoma: between one-third and two-thirds of patients have antibody to hepatitis C virus.

Sporadic infection: there is evidence that a small proportion of cases of sporadic hepatitis in the general population are due to hepatitis C.

Chronic active hepatitis: evidence of previous hepatitis C is present in a significant proportion of patients.

Virology

Little is known because the virus cannot be cultivated in cell culture. But it does infect chimpanzees and, by brilliant biotechnology, a virus-specific protein has been genetically engineered from virus in infected chimpanzee blood: this protein is the antigen in the newly developed test for anti-hepatitis C virus antibody.

1. Unclassified virus (possibly a flavivirus)
2. RNA genome—single-stranded, positive sense RNA
3. Does not grow in cell culture
4. Infects chimpanzees with production of viraemia.

Diagnosis

Still experimental but likely to become widely available—indicated especially for screening of donations for blood transfusion.

Serology: by ELISA and RIA: not useful for diagnosis of acute infection, as seroconversion is delayed: *note*: sera must not be heat-treated before test.

HEPATITIS D (DELTA AGENT)

This interesting virus—also known as delta agent—is defective and can only replicate in the presence of an appropriate helper virus which supplies the necessary gene product. The helper virus is hepatitis B so the hepatitis D virus is found only in patients infected with hepatitis B.

Pathogenicity: it is unclear what role the virus plays in liver disease: there is evidence that it increases the severity of—and may exacerbate attacks in the clinical course of—hepatitis B.

Epidemiology

Hepatitis D virus is found among drug abusers infected with hepatitis B—less often amongst other infected groups. The ecology of the virus is unknown—for example, it is unclear how the virus maintains itself in populations, from where it originated, and so on.

Virology

Little is known: the virus has a genome of single-stranded RNA and forms a small particle coated with HBsAg and 35–37 nm in diameter.

Diagnosis

Serology: ELISA test for antigen and antibody are available only on a research basis at a few specialist laboratories.

HEPATITIS E

Virtually nothing is known of the virology of hepatitis E. What is certain is that there is a form of hepatitis, seen in community outbreaks (sometimes very large) and apparently due to water-borne spread.

Incubation period: approximately 30–40 days.

Clinically: predominantly a disease of young adults, but of particular severity in pregnant women in whom high case fatality rates have been recorded.

Geographically: mainly seen in Asia, Africa and the Middle East. The extensive epidemic of water-borne hepatitis in Delhi in 1955 was probably due to hepatitis E.

Laboratory: no virological test is available.

15 Antiviral therapy

Antiviral drugs are available only for a minority of virus infections. Nevertheless, where appropriate, they are now making a significant impact on the management of virus disease. The number of effective antiviral drugs can be expected to increase in the future. The table below shows the main diseases for which effective therapy is available and the antiviral agents with which they can be treated.

Table 15.1 Antiviral therapy

Disease	Antiviral drug
Herpes simplex	Acyclovir, idoxuridine, vidarabine
Varicella-zoster	Acyclovir, idoxuridine, vidarabine
Cytomegalovirus	Ganciclovir
AIDS	Zidovudine
Respiratory syncytial virus, bronchiolitis or pneumonia	Ribavirin
Influenza	Amantadine

ACYCLOVIR

A breakthrough in antiviral therapy when introduced in 1982 because it is non-toxic to cells but extremely inhibitory to herpes simplex virus replication.

Viruses inhibited:

 (i) herpes simplex virus types 1 and 2
(ii) varicella-zoster—but less sensitive to the drug than herpes simplex virus.

Action: a nucleoside analogue that inhibits virus DNA synthesis: acyclovir is phosphorylated by herpes-specific thymidine kinase and is then inhibitory to the virus-specific enzyme, DNA polymerase. Cellular DNA polymerase is resistant to the inhibition and, since the drug is inactive unless in phosphorylated form, it is also inactive in uninfected cells and therefore virtually non-toxic.

Administration: oral, topical, intravenous (for severe infection).

Indications for use:

Treatment

1. Herpes simplex—for example, encephalitis, genital herpes, cold sores, dendritic ulcer of the cornea, herpes simplex in the immunocompromised
   Note: acyclovir does not eradicate latent virus so that reactivations are not prevented—although they may be suppressed by long term prophylaxis.
2. Varicella-zoster—severe varicella in leukaemic or other immunocompromised children; zoster—especially in the immunocompromised
   Note: acyclovir must be used in higher dosage than with herpes simplex.

Prophylaxis: prevents mucocutaneous reactivations of both herpes simplex and zoster in the immunocompromised (e.g. organ transplant recipients, leukaemia patients etc.).

Side-effects: usually minor: rashes, gastrointestinal disturbance, renal impairment—usually transient.

IDOXURIDINE

Severe side-effects have limited the use of this drug to topical application. It has largely been replaced by acyclovir.

Action: a nucleoside analogue which inhibits viral DNA synthesis

Indications for use: dendritic ulcer of cornea due to herpes simplex virus; occasionally, lesions of zoster and genital herpes.

Side-effects: not significant with topical application: but can cause severe bone marrow depression if used systemically.

VIDARABINE

Similar to idoxuridine in action and also associated with side-effects which are sometimes severe.

Administered: systemically by slow intravenous infusion.

Indications for use: varicella and zoster in the immunocompromised.

GANCICLOVIR

Also a nucleoside analogue and, as yet, of uncertain efficacy.

Administered: by slow intravenous infusion.

Indications for use: severe, life-threatening cytomegalovirus infections in the immunocompromised, e.g. pneumonia, retinitis.

Side-effects: neutropenia—and thrombocytopenia—are common: also, fever, rash, impaired renal function and abnormal liver function tests.

Foscarnet: also a DNA polymerase inhibitor, can be used to treat cytomegalovirus retinitis: administer by intravenous infusion. Renal toxicity may be a problem.

ZIDOVUDINE

Also a nucleoside analogue and, to date, the only specific antiviral therapy for HIV-infection. Of proven value in delaying death but does not eradicate infection or effect cure. Current trials are in progress to determine whether, if used before symptoms develop, the drug can prevent or delay onset of symptomatic AIDS or pre-AIDS.

Action: inhibits reverse transcriptase activity and so viral replication.

Administered: orally.

Side-effects: anaemia, bone marrow depression with neutropenia: hepatic and renal impairment.

RIBAVIRIN

A nucleoside analogue active against a wide range of viruses. Licensed in UK against severe respiratory syncytial virus infection but can also be used (if without certain efficacy proved in controlled trials) for severe virus diseases such as Lassa fever.

Action: inhibits viral nucleic acid replication.

Administered: by aerosol within a hood (this greatly limits its usefulness).

Indications for use: severe respiratory syncytial virus infection in infants, such as bronchiolitis, or bronchopneumonia.

Side-effects: reticulocytosis; respiratory depression.

AMANTADINE

Active against influenza A but not influenza B. It has been shown to be effective for both the treatment and prophylaxis of infection. It might prove invaluable in the face of an influenza A pandemic if sufficient vaccine could not be prepared in time to produce herd immunity. However, it has never been widely used.

Action: blocks penetration of virus into cells, probably with other antiviral activities also.

Administered: orally.

Indications for use: treatment and prevention of influenza A.

Side-effects: especially in the elderly, insomnia, nervousness, dizziness.

Note: amantadine is also used for zoster and post-herpetic neuralgia, but its efficacy is uncertain.

Inosine pranobex: can be used to treat mucocutaneous herpes simplex. It appears to stimulate the immune response, but its efficacy is uncertain. Administered orally.

INTERFERON

Although there were early reports to confirm, in human trials, that interferon (see Ch. 1) had antiviral activity, it has proved disappointing in practice. There is now evidence that interferon has a significant effect in clearing hepatitis *e* antigen and virus DNA in chronic hepatitis B infection. It is also used for AIDS-related Kaposi's sarcoma (and some other human cancers) and for condylomata acuminata. Surprisingly, since it is a substance secreted naturally in the body in response to viral and other stimuli, interferon therapy causes pyrogen-like side-effects, e.g. the symptoms of a 'flu-like' illness. Less often are anorexia, weight loss and symptoms of CNS disturbance.

16 Chronic neurological diseases due to viruses

Viruses can cause chronic disease of the CNS—also classified as 'slow virus diseases' (although some slow virus diseases are not neurological). These diseases have a long incubation period, slow development of symptoms and a protracted, but eventually fatal course. Some are chronic infections with conventional viruses but others are due to unconventional agents which may be viruses but are certainly quite unlike most human pathogenic viruses. Examples of such diseases in man due to conventional viruses are listed in Table 16.1. There are many examples in animals due to a variety of different viruses.

Table 16.1 Chronic neurological virus diseases due to conventional viruses

Virus	Disease
Measles	Subacute sclerosing panencephalitis
Rubella	Subacute sclerosing panencephalitis (follows congenital infection)
J C (human polyoma virus)	Progressive multifocal leucoencephalopathy

Subacute sclerosing panencephalitis has been described in Chapter 12. Progressive multifocal leucoencephalopathy is described below:

PROGRESSIVE MULTIFOCAL LEUCOENCEPHALOPATHY

This rare disease is due to a papovavirus known as JC, one of two known human polyoma viruses. The other is BK virus and is not neurotropic. JC virus is 'opportunistic' in that it only causes disease—as distinct from symptomless infection—in patients whose health is compromised by pre-existing disease such as a leukaemia or reticulosis or by immunosuppressive therapy.

Progressive multifocal leucoencephalopathy is due to reactivation of JC virus latent in the brain.

Clinical features

Varied neurological signs: such as hemiparesis, dementia, dysphasia, incoordination, impaired vision and hemianaesthesia.

Duration: usually fatal in 3 to 4 months.

Pathology: multiple foci of demyelination in cerebral hemispheres and cerebellum: brain stem and basal ganglia are also sometimes affected: oligodendrocytes with swollen nuclei and intranuclear inclusions are characteristic features.

Epidemiology

Infection with the virus is common in the community and around 50–60% of adults in Britain have antibody to it; it does not cause disease in normal people and progressive multifocal leucoencephalopathy is a rare complication due to reactivation of latent virus in an immunocompromised host.

Virology

1. Papovavirus—in the genus polyomavirus
2. Genome is circular, double-stranded DNA
3. Electron microscopy: small icosahedral particles with 72 capsomeres; size 42–45 nm
4. Grows in human fetal glial tissue cultures; virus growth is recognized by electron microscopy
5. Haemagglutinates human and guinea-pig erythrocytes at 4°C.

Note: the other human polyoma virus—BK virus—is also an opportunistic pathogen. It has been isolated from immunodeficient patients, mainly from urine (and sometimes with ureteric stenosis) due to reactivation of latent virus. Like JC virus, BK antibody is present in a proportion of human populations so that symptomless infection seems to be widespread. *Viruria* with both JC and BK virus is not uncommon in pregnancy—around 3–7% of pregnant women excrete human polyomaviruses.

Oncogenicity

Both JC and BK viruses transform cells in tissue culture in vitro.

NEUROLOGICAL VIRUS DISEASES DUE TO UNCONVENTIONAL AGENTS

There are three virus diseases, all of which involve the CNS, and which are due to unconventional agents. These are clearly not typical viruses and have never been seen in the electron microscope.

Infections with the agents show the following features:

1. Long incubation period
2. Protracted, severe, progressive course: virtually always fatal
3. Pathology: degeneration of the CNS with status spongiosus
4. Lesions show no inflammatory reaction
5. No antibody or other immune response.

Three diseases of this type are listed in Table 16.2.

Table 16.2   Chronic neurological diseases due to unconventional agents

Disease	Host species	Pathological features	Disease syndrome
Creutzfeldt-Jakob disease	Man	Subacute degeneration of brain and spinal cord with status spongiosus of cortex	Presenile dementia; ataxia, spasticity, involuntary movements
Kuru	Man	Subacute cerebellar degeneration; status spongiosus	Postural instability; ataxia, tremor
Scrapie	Sheep	Subacute cerebellar degeneration	Ataxia, tremor, constant rubbing; susceptibility to infection is genetically determined

Of these diseases, scrapie is the only one in which the causal agent has been subjected to intensive laboratory study. Even so, its nature and structure remain unknown.

SCRAPIE

Scrapie is a neurological disease common in Britain 200 years ago and now present in sheep in other countries also. It is clearly due to an infectious agent about the size of a small virus—possibly a prion (see below).

Clinical features

Natural scrapie affects both sheep and goats; the following are features of natural scrapie in sheep:

Long incubation period: from 2 to 5 years.

Signs and symptoms: affected sheep suffer from excitability, incoordination, ataxia, tremor and continuous scratching or rubbing due to sensory neurological disturbance; the symptoms progress to paralysis and death.

Pathology: cerebellar neuronal degeneration with astrocytic proliferation; status spongiosus—a vacuolating form of neuronal degeneration is a diagnostic feature.

Heredity: a major gene controls whether or not sheep develop disease after experimental inoculation; the operation of the gene is complex and depends partly on the strain of agent used for inoculation.

Route of infection: the disease is transmitted by contact in flocks of sheep and also vertically from ewes to lambs.

Scrapie agent

Scrapie can be transmitted by intracerebral or subcutaneous inoculation using the brains of infected sheep. The incubation period varies from 3 to 24 months depending on the strain of agent; the disease can also be transmitted to and passaged in mice in a shorter incubation period of 4 to 8 weeks; experimental infection in mice forms the basic technique of assaying the agent.

Properties

1. Small size—20 to 30 nm
2. Resistant to ultraviolet irradiation, formaldehyde and heat (e.g. resists 80°C for 60 minutes)
3. Does not stimulate antibody production in experimental animals.

No nucleic acid has been demonstrated in the scrapie agent nor has it been seen by electron microscopy; the remarkable resistance to ultraviolet irradiation suggests that if nucleic acid is present it must be in small amounts. Current evidence suggests that scrapie agent may be a *prion*—a postulated new class of agents which are infectious proteins. An altered host protein, PrP—or prion protein, is a characteristic feature of scrapie and is found in the brain and other tissues of affected animals.

BOVINE SPONGIFORM ENCEPHALOPATHY (BSE)

In the past few years, scrapie has been transmitted to cattle fed on feed containing sheep offal. The infection is now a major epidemic in the cattle herds of England and Wales. It is a cause of considerable concern that the agent of scrapie could so rapidly cross a species barrier to cause an epidemic in cattle. So far there is no evidence of similar spread to humans.

TRANSMISSIBLE MINK ENCEPHALOPATHY

A disease also spread from sheep products and due to scrapie agent: mink bred in mink farms become infected when fed on the heads of scrapie-infected sheep.

CREUTZFELDT-JAKOB DISEASE

A rare progressive neurological disease characterized by a combination of presenile symptoms due to lesions in the spinal cord.

Clinical features

1. *Prodromal stage*: the disease starts with tiredness, apathy and vague neurological symptoms
2. *Second stage*: the patients develop ataxia, dysarthria and progressive spasticity of the limbs; this is associated with

dementia and often involutary movements such as myoclonic jerks or choreo-athetoid movements
3. *The disease progresses steadily* until death—usually from about six months to two years after the onset of symptoms
4. *Pathology*: diffuse atrophy with status spongiosus in the cerebral cortex; atrophy also in basal ganglia, cerebellum, substantia nigra and anterior horn cells.

Causal agent

Transmission experiments: the disease is reproduced in chimpanzees and other primates after intracerebral inoculation of brain tissues from cases of the disease; the incubation period is from 11 to 14 months; the disease can also be transmitted peripherally (by combined intravenous, intraperitoneal and intramuscular routes).

Human infection: the natural route of infection is unknown but Creutzfeldt-Jakob disease has been accidently transmitted via a corneal graft to the recipient. Transmissions have also been reported from a patient with the disease to other patients by electrodes used for electro-encephalography. Recently, transmission of the disease has been reported in patients injected with growth hormone derived from human pituitary gland and in two patients who received grafts of dura mater from cadavers.

Gerstmann-Sträussler-Scheinker's disease: is a similar but atypical form of Creutzfeldt-Jakob disease also transmissible to primates. There is some evidence of inherited familial susceptibility.

Note: Chronic neurological disease due to unconventional agents has attracted considerable interest because of the possibility that human neurological diseases of unknown cause (e.g. multiple sclerosis, motor neurone disease, and Alzheimer's disease) might be due to similar agents.

KURU

Kuru is a fatal human disease found only among the Foré-speaking people in New Guinea. It seems to have appeared about 60 years ago. The incidence increased up until the late 1950s when kuru was responsible for about half the deaths in the Foré-speaking people. The incidence of kuru has now declined rapidly since the early 1960s.

Clinical features

Kuru is a native word meaning 'trembling with cold and fever'.

Incubation period: around 4 to 20 years.

The first or ambulant stage of the disease starts with unsteadiness in walking, postural instability, ataxia and tremor; facial expressions are poorly controlled and speech becomes slurred and tremulous.

The second or sedentary stage is reached when the patient cannot walk without support, but can still sit upright unaided.

In the tertiary stage the patient cannot sit upright without clutching a stick for support; even a gentle push makes the patient lurch violently; the patient becomes progressively more paralysed and emaciated until death, which is due to bulbar depression or intercurrent infection.

Duration of the disease averages one year but ranges from three months to two years.

Pathology: neuronal degeneration in cerebellum with astrocytic hyperplasia, gliosus and status spongiosus; demyelination is minimal or absent.

Epidemiology

Sex incidence: kuru is uncommon in adult males; most patients are women or children of both sexes.

Cannibalism of dead relatives is thought to have been responsible for the spread of kuru among the Foré people. The women and children (but not men) eat the viscera and brains of relatives including those who have died of kuru. Spread may have been through contact of infected tissues with abrasions on skin rather than, or as well as, ingestion. The tissues are inadequately cooked so the causal agent would not be inactivated by cooking.

Cannibalism stopped around 1957 and kuru has now declined sharply in incidence.

Transmission experiments: intracerebral inoculation of brain tissue from kuru victims into chimpanzees and other primates causes the animals to develop the symptoms of kuru after an incubation period of two years.

17 Warts

Warts are one of the commonest virus infections and few people reach adult life without suffering from them. The extensive—albeit still incomplete—knowledge of their virology is a tribute to modern biotechnology since cultivation in vitro has never been achieved.

Clinical features

Warts: are benign tumours of the skin with virus-induced proliferation of keratinized and non-keratinized squamous epithelium—i.e. both skin and mucous membranes.

Most common on hands and feet, warts also infect the genitalia and anus where they may be large and known as condylomata acuminata; recent evidence suggests that small, clinically symptomless warts are common in the female population: warts are also found in the larynx and oral cavity.

Table 17.1 lists the principal clinical types of wart and the papilloma viruses found in them.

Condylomata acuminata: a common—and increasing—sexually transmitted disease: occasionally very large (Plate 6): rarely, and apparently only in immunocompromised women, the warts have become malignant with change to invasive squamous epithelioma.

Laryngeal papilloma: rare in Britain, but relatively common in other countries, e.g. southern United States: the juvenile form is acquired during birth from maternal condylomata acuminata: laryngeal warts show a marked tendency to recur after treatment.

Epidermodysplasia verruciformis: a rare autosomal recessive inherited disease in which affected patients develop multiple

Table 17.1   Main types of wart and the human papillomaviruses with which they are associated

Wart	Papillomavirus type
Plantar	1, 4
Hand	2
Flat; juvenile	3, 10
Condylomata acuminata	6, 11, 16
Carcinoma of cervix	16, 18
Laryngeal	6, 11, 30
Warts and macules in epidermodysplasia verruciformis	5, 8, (and other types not found in other warts)
Butcher's warts	7

warts with a high risk (around one-third) of malignant change to squamous cell carcinomas. Interestingly, the papillomaviruses responsible for the warts seem to belong to several different and unusual types of virus: types 5 and 8 papillomaviruses are the commonest found in the lesions.

Butcher's warts: are an occupational hazard of slaughtermen and butchers: due to type 7 virus which is not found in human populations and for which to date, no animal source has been detected.

Epidemiology

Spread: by contact, e.g. hand to hand; via water in the surrounds of swimming pools in the case of plantar warts on the feet; sexual transmission in genital warts and via the birth canal with juvenile laryngeal papillomas.

Ecology: this is still unclear.

Papillomaviruses and cancer

There is strong evidence that papillomaviruses can, although perhaps not without a co-factor, transform or cause cells to become malignant. Amongst animals (many, perhaps all, species of which have their own host-specific papillomaviruses) some of the viruses cause cancer. In American cotton tailrabbits, the Shope papilloma which is virus-induced becomes cancerous in 25% of animals: in domestic rabbits, similar experimentally-induced Shope papillomas undergo malignant change at a much higher rate. Amongst cattle, alimentary papillomas—due to bovine papilloma virus type 4—became malignant when the animals were fed on bracken.

Human cancer

There is good evidence that papillomaviruses cause human cancer. This is based on three main observations:

1. The frequent malignant change in virus-induced warts in epidermodysplasia verruciformis
2. The—admittedly rare—development of cancer in vulvar warts in women with lymphoma
3. The frequent association of papillomavirus type 18 DNA (and, less often, that of type 16) with invasive cervical cancer.

Cervical cancer

Cervical cancer shows epidemiological characteristics which suggest it might be due to a sexually-transmitted agent. For example, it shows strong risk factors such as early age at first intercourse, multiple sexual partners, high parity etc.: the disease in fact correlates with high sexual activity: it is virtually unknown in nuns. The disease is preceded in the majority of cases by pre-cancerous or early malignant lesions known as cervical intraepithelial neoplasia (CIN) formerly called carcinoma-in-situ. These pre-malignant lesions of CIN contain DNA of papillomaviruses types 6 and 11—less often that of type 16.

Small, symptomless cervical warts are surprisingly common in women. The less common and larger condylomata acuminata consistently contain DNA of types 6 and 11. In contrast, types 16 and 18 can regularly be detected in invasive cervical carcinoma, although type 18 is not found in pre-malignant CIN. It can, therefore, be concluded that papillomaviruses are found consistently in a high proportion of cervical cancers, although not necessarily of the same type as that found in pre-malignant lesions. Clearly, new research is required to elucidate the pathogenesis—and the role of papillomavirus in it—of cervical cancer.

Skin cancer

Squamous cell carcinomas develop relatively frequently in the warts associated with epidermodysplasia verruciformis: these warts are due to papillomaviruses types 5 and 8. Interestingly, warts are common in patients with renal transplants; in these patients (who are, of course, immunocompromised) there is a high risk of squamous cell cancer—again associated with types 5 and 8 papillomaviruses.

Virology

1. Papovavirus family; papillomavirus genus: 56 types have been identified on the basis of DNA homology

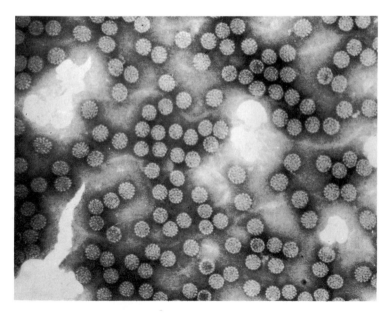

Fig. 17.1   Human papillomavirus. The virus particles have cubic symmetry. × 90 000. (Photograph by Dr E. A. C. Follett.)

2. DNA virus—with double-stranded, circular DNA
3. Electron microscopy: icosahedral particle with 72 capsomeres, 52–55 nm in diameter (Fig. 17.1)
4. Host-specific: do not grow in any cell cultures: not pathogenic for any non-human animals.

Diagnosis

The virus DNA can be demonstrated in tissue by radioactive DNA probe: this is used for experimental and research purposes.

Typing

Papillomaviruses are typed by estimation of the degree of DNA homology by hybridization of their DNA with that of other well-characterized human papillomaviruses.

18 Retroviruses

The discovery of human retroviruses has been one of the most important developments in clinical virology in recent years. Long known as the cause of natural cancer in various animal species, retrovirus research has led to major advances in knowledge of the molecular basis of cancer.

ANIMAL RETROVIRUSES

Many retroviruses cause natural cancer in the host animal. They also produce tumours—which are mainly leukaemia or sarcomas —on inoculation into experimental animals. Although sarcoma viruses transform cells most of the leukaemia viruses do not.

Morphology

Retroviruses have similar but also slightly different types of particle:

1. C-type particles: most retroviruses have spherical enveloped particles surrounded by spikes or knobs and containing a central core composed of RNA and protein (Fig. 18.1)
2. B-type particles: mouse mammary tumour virus (also a retrovirus) has particles similar to C-type particles but with an eccentric core or nucleoid.
3. D-type particles: have typical retrovirus morphology but with a central cylindrical core, and are typified by HIV—the virus of human acquired immune deficiency syndrome (AIDS)—and also by Mason-Pfizer Monkey virus.

Note: All retrovirus particles contain the enzyme reverse transcriptase (see Ch. 2).

155

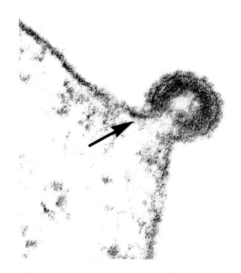

Fig. 18.1   Feline leukaemia virus—a typical C-type retrovirus particle budding through the plasma membrane on its release from the cell. The continuity between the cell surface membrane and the virion is indicated by the arrow and the spikes on the surface of the outer virion membrane are clearly seen × 190 000. (Photograph by Helen Laird.)

Genome structure

The retrovirus genome is diploid consisting of two identical molecules in inverse orientation. There are three main genes:

1. The *gag* gene—codes for the core protein antigens of the virus particle. These are cleaved from a larger precursor protein
2. The *pol* gene—codes for the protein that is the reverse transcriptase
3. The *env* gene—codes for the glycoprotein envelope proteins of the virion.

Long terminal repeat regions: at each end of the genome contain powerful promoter and enhancer sequences: responsible for the integration of provirus—the DNA transcript of the genome RNA produced by reverse transcriptase—into cellular chromosome.

Additional genes: tat (transactivating transcription), *trs*, *lor*, etc. have been described in the human retroviruses.

Oncogenes

Many retrovirus genomes contain oncogenes incorporated into

their structure. Oncogenes are genes whose expression is associated with tumour production. It is now clear that oncogenes are present as a result of vertical inheritance in many normal cells. Retroviruses cause cancer when their genome acquires cellular oncogenes by recombination. This probably happens when RNA tumour viruses integrate in the form of provirus DNA into cellular chromosomes. Numerous oncogenes have been described in animal retroviruses. In these cases their designation is preceded by the letter 'v' e.g. v-*myc* or v-*ras*: their cellular counterparts are known as c-*myc* or c-*ras*. Activated cellular oncogenes may differ by only a single base mutation from their normal progenitor gene. Oncogenes do not always give rise to carcinogenesis. They need to be activated and different mechanisms can be responsible for this:

1. A virus promoter such as that contained in the long terminal repeat regions of the retrovirus genome.
2. A cellular promoter—possibly by translocation of the oncogene to a site on a chromosome with high activity.
3. A co-factor such as a chemical carcinogen
4. Interaction with other oncogenes.

It seems likely that oncogenes normally function as regulatory mechanisms in cells: their activation to produce tumours is probably the result of a loss of control of normal gene function leading to disturbance of the usual regulatory activity.

Epidemiology

Most animal species (including man) in which a detailed search has been made are natural hosts for retroviruses that are characteristic of the species.

Transmission

Transmission from animal to animal takes place in three ways:

1. *Horizontal*: in which the virus spreads by direct contact, or possibly inhalation, between infected and susceptible animals. This is an important route in naturally-occurring infection in outbred animals not reared in a laboratory, such as cats.
2. *Congenital*: vertical transmission in which the virus spreads from mother to offspring either by infection in utero or via the mother's milk.

3. *Genetic*: also vertical transmission but in this case the virus is inherited in the form of a provirus or viral DNA transcript integrated into the chromosomes of the germ cells of the parent animal. The viruses produced from proviruses are known as *endogenous* viruses and are typical retroviruses: however, although some are tumour-producing on inoculation into experimental animals, many are not. Endogenous retroviruses are usually present in a repressed state but can be induced by various agents so that their genes are derepressed with consequent production of the virus in the animal.

Endogenous retroviruses are present in normal cells of chickens, mice, cats and primates. Retrovirus sequences have been identified in human chromosomes.

TUMOURS PRODUCED BY RETROVIRUSES

Most retroviruses which cause tumours in animals can be divided into:

1. sarcoma viruses
2. leukaemia viruses.

Sarcoma viruses

Sarcoma viruses readily transform cells in tissue culture and produce solid tumours—fibrosarcomas—on inoculation into animals of the host species. Most are defective so that, in order to replicate, they require the presence of a helper virus (usually a leukaemia virus of the same animal species) to supply the product of the defective gene. The defective viruses have deletions in one or more of the three structural genes, because host genes with oncogenic potential have been substituted in their place. The deletion often involves the *env* gene and as a result sarcoma viruses are serologically related—with the same type-specific neutralizing antigen in their envelope—to the helper leukaemia virus.

Leukaemia viruses

Leukaemia viruses produce leukaemia on inoculation into animals. Many do not transform cells in tissue culture although some do so. Leukaemia viruses are not defective and generally replicate in tissue culture. They do not produce CPE and cell growth and division are not affected.

Table 18.1 lists the principle tumour-producing animal retroviruses, their host animal species and the tumours produced.

Table 18.1   Animal tumour-producing retroviruses

Host animal	Virus	Tumour
Chickens	Rous sarcoma virus Avian leukosis viruses	Sarcoma in chickens Fowl leukaemia
Mice	Murine sarcoma virus Murine leukaemia viruses Mouse mammary tumour virus	Sarcoma in mice Mouse leukaemia Breast cancer in mice
Cats	Feline sarcoma virus Feline leukaemia virus	Sarcoma in cats Cat leukaemia
Primates	Simian sarcoma virus Gibbon ape leukaemia virus	Sarcoma in marmosets Leukaemia in gibbon apes

HUMAN RETROVIRUSES

Four have been discovered: they are listed below in Table 18.2. All are lymphotropic for $CD4^+$ carrying or T4 lymphocytes, but whereas HTLV-1 and 2 transform and cause T4 lymphocytes to proliferate, HIV-1 and 2 are cytopathic and kill the cells. The CD4 receptors on the lymphocytes are the receptors for the viruses.

Table 18.2   Human retroviruses

Virus	Disease
Human T-cell lymphotropic virus Type 1(HTLV-1) Type 2(HTLV-2)	T-cell leukaemia/lymphoma: tropical spastic paraparesis Unknown
Human immunodeficiency virus Type 1 (HIV-1) Type 2 (HIV-2)	Acquired immune deficiency syndrome (AIDS) AIDS

HTLV-1

HTLV-1 is an endemic infection particularly prevalent in south-western Japan and in the Caribbean, where it causes adult T-cell leukaemia/lymphoma. Elsewhere, leukaemia/lymphoma is predominantly a tumour of B lymphocytes. More recently the virus has been found to cause tropical spastic paraparesis or, as it is called in Japan, HTLV-1-associated myelopathy.

Clinical features

T-cell leukaemia/lymphoma: an aggressive malignancy of T4 lymphocytes, with lymphadenopathy and hepatosplenomegaly; cerebral involvement is common. The disease often presents with lymphomatous infiltration of the skin (so that it can be mistaken clinically for mycosis fungoides): characteristically there is an increased level of calcium in the blood, which may be related to osteoporotic lesions in bones—another characteristic feature.

Tropical spastic paraparesis: a progressive, non-demyelinating spastic paralysis, more common in females than males.

Symptomless infection: is common and the risk factors that lead to the onset of disease are unknown. The majority of those infected do not develop disease.

Virus is present as a latent infection in the T-lymphocytes of infected individuals. In patients with T-cell leukaemia/lymphoma, atypical transformed T-lymphocytes are present, sometimes in large numbers, in the peripheral blood.

Antibody persists throughout the infection: titres are variable but are high in patients with tropical spastic paraparesis.

Epidemiology

Geographical distribution: marked; infection is particularly common in southwestern Japan, the Caribbean and West Africa. It is also present in Britain, mostly in immigrants from the West Indies.

Spread: via blood, but since the virus is markedly cell-associated it is not transmitted via plasma products; breast milk (therefore from mother to child).

Seroprevalence: antibody to HTLV-1 is endemic, reaching a prevalence of 10% in the populations most affected. The prevalence of antibody in children is low, but rises with increasing age in adult life.

Virology

1. Retrovirus; oncornavirus
2. RNA virus with typical retrovirus genome structure
3. Electron microscopy—C-type particles: the particles contain reverse transcriptase
4. Grows in culture in human T-lymphocytes stimulated with interleukin 2: cells are transformed or immortalized: there is no cytopathic effect.

Diagnosis

Serology: RIA, ELISA and immunofluorescence tests, but these are available at only a few research centres.

HTLV-2

Originally isolated from a patient with hairy cell leukaemia, the virus is now thought to be unrelated to this disease. Similar structurally and with extensive nucleic acid homology to HTLV-1, its pathogenicity is unknown. Small clusters of antibody-positive people have been described amongst drug abusers in London and in several cities in the USA.

HIV

The cause of AIDS and presently the most intensively-investigated virus of all. AIDS results from a collapse of the immune system, triggered off by, and also largely due to, the cytopathic effect of HIV on T4 helper lymphocytes. Note that some animal retroviruses, for example, some variants of feline leukaemia virus, also cause immunodeficiency. The human disease is unusual in that it appears to be a genuinely new disease. The first infection recorded was in Kinshasa, Zaire, in 1959 (where antibody to HIV was later detected in a serum taken at that time). However, it remains uncertain whether HIV originated in Africa. Since then, AIDS has become epidemic in Africa and, with a somewhat different epidemiology, in the USA and Western Europe and has now been found in virtually every country in the world.

HIV: there are two types of virus—HIV-1 the main cause of the worldwide AIDS pandemic and HIV-2, recently discovered in West Africa and, as yet, not showing significant spread from there.

Clinical features

Four groups of clinical features are associated with the progression of HIV infection.

First, seen some 14 days after infection, an infectious mononucleosis-like illness with fever, sore throat, night sweats, malaise, lymphadenopathy, diarrhoea, and relative and absolute lymphocytosis in the peripheral blood. There may be mouth and genital ulcers. The symptoms subside spontaneously, and antibody appears about this time.

Second: a variable symptomless period, usually round 2–7 years, during which some patients show depressed counts of T4 lymphocytes.

Third: persistent generalized lymphadenopathy with reappearance of symptoms—notably enlarged lymph nodes at two or more extra-inguinal sites which persist for at least three months. These signs are often, although not inevitably, a prelude to progression to full-blown AIDS. Opportunistic infections may begin to appear at this stage—most often with diarrhoea, wasting and oral candidiasis.

Progression to AIDS correlates with decrease in T4 lymphocyte count, the appearance of the internal core antigen, P24, in the blood and fall in titre of anti-P24 antibody.

Fourth: Full-blown AIDS is characterized by an extreme degree of immunodeficiency. This results in a series of opportunistic infections as micro-organisms, uncontrolled by the patient's immune mechanisms, proliferate to cause a variety of unusually severe infections. It is now clear that AIDS has other features in addition to infection with secondary opportunistic pathogens.

AIDS is a syndrome with the following features:

A. *Constitutional disease*: fever, diarrhoea, weight loss
B. *Neurological disease*: dementia, sometimes myelopathy or peripheral neuropathy
C. *Secondary infectious diseases*: opportunistic infections (see Table 18.3 but, note, a variety of other infections are also seen)
D. *Secondary cancers* (see below)
E. *Other conditions.*

'Unique' features: AIDS has an extraordinarily wide variety of associated signs and symptoms. None are absolutely pathognomonic of the disease, but two diseases are particularly characteristic and should always raise suspicion of AIDS:

(i) Kaposi's sarcoma
(ii) hairy leukoplakia of the tongue.

Table 18.3   Infections associated with AIDS

Infectious agent	Disease
Parasites	
Pneumocystis carinii	Pneumonia
Cryptosporidium	Diarrhoea
Isospora belli	Diarrhoea
Strongyloides stercoralis	Diarrhoea
Toxoplasma gondii	Encephalitis
	Chorioretinitis
Viruses	
Herpes simplex	Oral ulceration
Cytomegalovirus	Pneumonia
	Retinitis
JC virus	Progressive multifocal leucoencephalopathy
Bacteria	
Mycobacterium avium-intracellulare	Respiratory disease
	Disseminated infection
Mycobacterium tuberculosis	Tuberculosis
Salmonella spp	Diarrhoea
Fungi	
Candida albicans	Oral ulceration, oesophagitis
Cryptococcus neoformans	Pneumonia, meningitis

Note: Many of these infections are severe, with a tendency to cause disseminated infection not seen in immunocompetent people

Non-specific signs and symptoms: patients are anaemic with high erythrocyte sedimentation rate: rashes and dry flaky skin with itching: persistent diarrhoea: myalgia and arthralgia; sometimes snuffles, sore throat, headache.

T-lymphocyte destruction is a cardinal sign of AIDS: T4 (helper T-lymphocytes) are severely depleted with consequent distortion of the normal helper/suppressor T-cell ratio.

In Africa weight loss is a prominent symptom, so that AIDS has been called 'slim disease'.

A progressive dementia is now recognized as a feature of AIDS and due to direct virus infection of the brain. This can take many forms—principally dementia but also depression, personality change, convulsions: cerebral atrophy is detected on CAT scanning.

Cancer: AIDS is also characterized by the unusual cancer, Kaposi's sarcoma. Kaposi's sarcoma is a cancer of the endothelial cells which line blood vessels but which appears as purplish tumours in the skin (Plate 7). As an AIDS-related tumour, Kaposi's sarcoma is much more aggressive and more rapidly fatal than when it is unrelated to AIDS. This latter form is a rather indolent disease seen mainly, although relatively rarely, in African and some Mediterranean men. Kaposi's sarcoma in AIDS is seen predominantly in homosexual men.

Lymphoma: is also more common in AIDS patients, particularly cerebral lymphoma—a diagnostic feature of AIDS.

Note: AIDS is often described as a disease of T4 helper lymphocytes and although these are clearly major targets for the virus (which attaches specifically to the CD4 receptors on these and cells such as macrophages), it is becoming obvious that the virus causes disseminated infection and attacks many other types of cell and organs in the body. Much more research is needed into the pathogenicity of HIV infection.

HIV-2: is endemic, and spreading, in some countries in West Africa. So far it is rare in other parts of the world, although some cases of infection have been described in Portugal and France and amongst West African nationals in London. HIV-2 also causes AIDS, but disease associated with HIV-2 is generally milder than that associated with HIV-1.

Paediatric AIDS

Infected mothers: transmit HIV to their babies in approximately a third of cases: the virus may spread to the child either,

(i) transplacentally—to cause infection in utero
(ii) during delivery or in the perinatal period through breast feeding or close contact.

Clinically infected infants show the following signs and symptoms:

Failure to thrive
Fever
Diarrhoea
Frequent infections including opportunistic and disseminated infections
Lymphadenopathy
Lymphoid interstitial pneumonia
Parotitis
Hepatosplenomegaly
Neurological disease: most often a progressive encephalopathy, sometimes dementia, convulsions, motor disorders.

Paediatric AIDS: although broadly similar to adult AIDS, lymphoid interstitial pneumonia and parotid gland enlargement are not seen in the adult disease.

Infections: Candidiasis is very common. Paediatric infections like otitis media, staphylococcal infections (often invasive) and infections due to Gram-negative bacilli are frequent.

Serology: laboratory tests for HIV-specific IgM are not generally available, although specimens can be tested for this in specialized reference laboratories. The antibody detected in infants may be passively-transferred maternal IgG, but antibody persistence after 15 months of age is evidence that the child has become infected: however, some infected children do not develop antibody and others become antibody negative for a time before antibody reappears and persists.

Prognosis: most young children die within 1 year of a diagnosis of AIDS; but HIV infection in haemophiliac children progresses much more slowly with, in most cases, a prolonged period of symptomless infection.

Risk factors

The risk of heterosexual, non-drug abusing, formerly healthy individuals in Britain developing AIDS is low: AIDS is strongly associated with certain risk factors which reflect the mode of spread of the virus. These are listed in Table 18.4.

Table 18.4   Risk factors in AIDS

Male homosexuality

Haemophilia

Intravenous drug abuse

Prostitution

Sexual contact with
infected partner

Sexual contact in Africa

Transfusion with unscreened blood

Child of infected (or high risk) mother

Epidemiology

Sources of virus are infected body fluids, notably blood, semen and vaginal secretions. Saliva, although containing virus, is probably not a source of infection. The role of breast milk is also doubtful.

Route of infection: is mainly by *sexual intercourse*, but also parenterally by blood and blood products and sharing of syringes by drug abusers; rarely, needlestick injury with blood-contaminated needle.

In sub-Saharan Africa where the infection is now a major epidemic, spread is predominantly heterosexual with equal numbers of men and women infected.

In USA and Western Europe AIDS and HIV-1 infections are principally seen among homosexual men. But this is changing and, as HIV-1 infection spreads to drug abusers through the use of shared syringes, a higher proportion of women can be expected to become infected. Drug abusers can also become sources of spread through heterosexual contact. In Scotland, where HIV was introduced to the drug-abusing population at an early stage in the epidemic, around 30% of those infected are young women.

Haemophiliacs: about a third of haemophiliacs in Britain are infected with HIV-1, due to contamination with virus of some batches of Factor VIII which, before 1984, were not heat-treated. Blood transfusion is now not a source of infection as all donations are screened for HIV-1 antibody: before screening an occasional case of HIV-1 infection was traced to blood transfusion.

Geographical distribution: AIDS is now a worldwide disease, but is a far more serious problem in Africa than elsewhere. In several countries in Africa, a significant proportion (e.g. from 5–10%) of the adult population is infected with HIV.

Virology

1. Retrovirus: oncornavirus
2. RNA virus with genome structure as described above
   Note: the *env* gene, which codes for the main envelope glycoprotein, shows a considerable degree of spontaneous variation
3. Electron microscopy: D-type retrovirus particle
4. Grows in lymphocyte cultures, but without cytopathic effect. Co-cultivation with certain other cells results in syncytium formation and allows detection of virus growth
5. There is evidence that some features of AIDS can be reproduced by experimental inoculation of certain primates.

Diagnosis

Serology: ELISA test: if positive, confirm by *Western Blot* to analyse antibodies against virus structural proteins. HIV-1 and HIV-2 infections can be distinguished (although with some difficulty) by serological tests.

Demonstration of virus products

(i) *Antigen*: detect by ELISA in blood, other body fluids
(ii) *Reverse transcriptase*: assay can be used as a measure of virion-associated enzyme activity and, therefore, a crude indication of virus titre.

Treatment

Specific antiviral therapy: the drug *Zidovudine* inhibits virus replication by acting on viral reverse transcriptase. It prolongs survival and a recent report has indicated that it has some effect in preventing the onset of symptoms in infected, asymptomatic patients. However, it does not seem to alter the eventual fatal outcome. (See Ch. 15.)

Anti-infective therapy: Patients should also be treated with appropriate therapy for the opportunistic infections of AIDS as they arise.

VIRUSES AND CANCER

It has been known for many years that viruses can cause cancer. Experimentally, this oncogenicity can be demonstrated by:

(i) production of tumours on inoculation of virus into animals
(ii) transformation of normal cells in culture into cells with malignant characteristics.

However, many of the viruses which are oncogenic in the laboratory do not cause cancer naturally in their host animal. Despite much research, it has taken a long time to prove a viral cause for a human cancer. Although viruses are now known to be associated with some tumours, most human cancers have not been attributed to viruses.

Table 18.5 lists viruses known or strongly. suspected to cause human cancer; it includes both DNA and RNA viruses.

Table 18.5   Viruses and human cancer

Virus	Tumour
HTLV-1	T-cell leukaemia/lymphoma
Hepatitis B	Primary hepatocellular cancer
Papillomavirus	Squamous epithelioma development in some warts (Possibly) cervical, other genital cancers
Epstein-Barr virus	Burkitt's lymphoma; nasopharyngeal carcinoma; some lymphomas in the immunocompromised

19 Chlamydial diseases

Chlamydia are widespread in human and animal populations. They are not viruses although, by tradition, they are usually handled in virus laboratories. They are really bacteria but differ from bacteria in being unable to grow on inanimate media. They are sensitive to tetracycline and erythromycin.

There are three species of *Chlamydia*:

1. *Chlamydia trachomatis*
2. *Chlamydia pneumoniae*
3. *Chlamydia psittaci.*

Below in Table 19.1, are listed their serotypes and associated diseases.

Table 19.1   Chlamydia

Species	Hosts	Main diseases	Serotypes
Chlamydia trachomatis	Man	Oculogenital	D, E, F, G, H, I, J, K
		Trachoma Lymphogranuloma venereum	A, B, Ba, C. 1, 2, 3
Chlamydia pneumoniae		Pneumonia	—
Chlamydia psittaci	Various animals (including birds)	Psittacosis	—

Bacteriology of chlamydia

1. Contain both DNA and RNA
2. Larger than most viruses, 250-500 nm: visible by light microscopy

3. Replicate only within living cells: the growth cycle is complex and includes a stage of binary fusion
4. Grow in tissue culture: in McCoy or HeLa cells treated with cycloheximide or idoxuridine to stop cell division: chlamydial growth is recognized by intracytoplasmic inclusions detected by immunofluorescence (best with monoclonal antibody) or —less effective—by Giemsa staining
5. Grow in yolk sac of chick embryos
6. Sensitive to antibiotics, tetracycline, erythromycin, sulphonamides.

CHLAMYDIA TRACHOMATIS

Serotypes D to K of *Chlam. trachomatis* are widespread as causes of genital infection in human populations, generally transmitted by sexual intercourse. Infection of women is usually symptomless but, in men, they are responsible for the majority of cases of non-specific genital infection. These serotypes also cause eye disease and pneumonia. Another sexually transmitted disease seen in tropical countries—lymphogranuloma venereum—is due to serotypes 1, 2 and 3. Other serotypes cause trachoma, a serious eye infection in tropical countries.

Types D to K Non-specific genital infection

Also known as non-specific urethritis and by far the commonest sexually-transmitted disease in Britain.

Clinical features

Males: acute urethritis with urethral discharge, frequency, dysuria: there may be cystitis, epididymitis and prostatitis—or proctitis in homosexual males. Reiter's syndrome (a triad of urethritis, arthritis and conjunctivitis) is seen in a small proportion (less than 1%) of cases.

Females: infection commonly involves the cervix. Usually symptomless but sometimes accompanied by mild vaginitis with discharge. *Chlam. trachomatis* can cause salpingitis and pelvic inflammatory disease.

Treatment: Tetracycline, erythromycin.

Ocular infection

Chlam. trachomatis causes three types of eye infection:

(i) Neonatal ophthalmia
(ii) Inclusion conjunctivitis
(iii) Trachoma (see below).

Neonatal ophthalmia and inclusion conjunctivitis are seen in countries with a temperate climate, such as Britain: trachoma is a disease of tropical countries and is due to different serotypes.

Neonatal ophthalmia

Also called inclusion blennorrhoea. Seen in babies born to mothers with cervicitis as a result of contamination acquired during passage through the infected birth canal.

Clinically: a mucopurulent conjunctivitis appearing 1-2 weeks after birth.

Treatment: oral erythromycin.

Inclusion conjunctivitis

A disease mainly of children but sometimes of adults also. Probably acquired by indirect contact from genital infection: outbreaks have been reported amongst children at swimming baths (swimming pool conjunctivitis).

Clinically: a follicular conjunctivitis with mucopurulent discharge: chlamydial eye infection can cause punctate keratitis in which there is corneal involvement.

Treatment: oral tetracycline, erythromycin

3. Pneumonia

Chlam. trachomatis is now known to be a cause of pneumonia in neonates. Although conjunctivitis is a more common manifestation, pneumonia is seen in about a fifth of infected infants.

Clinically: often preceded by upper respiratory symptoms: the pneumonia is relatively mild with dry spasmodic cough and rapid breathing: the infants are not usually febrile. Chest X-rays show diffuse infiltration of the lungs.

Treatment: erythromycin.

Trachoma Types A to C

A major cause of blindness in the world and a scourge of tropical countries: tragically, a cause of needless suffering as it responds well to treatment: spread is from case to case by contact, contaminated fomites and flies.

Clinically: a severe follicular conjunctivitis with pannus (i.e. invasion of the cornea by blood vessels (Plate 8): corneal scarring which results in blindness is a common sequel.

Treatment: topical or oral tetracycline.

Lymphogranuloma venereum: types 1, 2, 3

A disease which is common in tropical countries but almost unknown in temperate climates. Cases in Britain are rare and the infection has usually been acquired abroad: the disease is generally sexually-transmitted.

Clinically: in males, the primary lesion is a painless ulcer on the penis which is often unnoticed. The disease then takes the form of the *inguinal syndrome* in which there is a painful enlargement of the inguinal and femoral lymph nodes which later may suppurate to form buboes. The *genito-anorectal syndrome* is the most common disease in women: infection involves the vagina and cervix—usually without symptoms—but the infection can then spread via the lymphatics to the rectum causing proctitis with bleeding and purulent discharge from the anus.

Treatment: Sulphonamides or tetracycline.

Diagnosis

Isolation

Specimens: genital or eye swabs; sputum.

Culture: in McCoy or HeLa cells.

Observe: for typical intracytoplasmic inclusions by immunofluorescence with monoclonal antibody—or Giemsa stain.

Direct demonstration

Specimens: swabs, smears from lesions.

Examine: by ELISA or by specific immunofluorescence of the typical intracytoplasmic inclusions—preferably with monoclonal antibody.

Serology (less useful)

1. *Micro-immunofluorescence tests* are type-specific so that sera must be tested against the appropriate range of serotypes (i.e. D, E, F, G, H, I, J, K for most chlamydial infections in Britain).
   IgM tests for the presence of IgM antibody can be used as an indicator of recent infection: detected by micro-immunofluorescence test.

2. *Complement fixation tests*: less sensitive than immunofluorescence tests. Chlamydiae share a common group complement fixing antigen so that it is only necessary to use one strain as antigen.

CHLAMYDIA PNEUMONIAE

Recently recognized as a cause of respiratory infection in human populations: mild or symptomless infection is probably quite common.

Chlam. pneumoniae (formerly called TWAR, i.e. Taiwan acute respiratory agent).

Clinical features

Respiratory: *Chlam. pneumoniae* has been recently found as a a cause of acute respiratory infection—typically a mild pneumonia but also sore throat with hoarseness, cough and fever.

Outbreaks: of pneumonia have been reported.

Epidemiology

Little is known but antibodies show quite a high prevalence in British communities studied.

Diagnosis

At present facilities for this are limited to a few centres. It seems certain that these will rapidly become available on a wider basis in the near future.

Serology: detection of antibody by micro-immunofluorescence but antibody is produced late after primary infection.

CHLAMYDIA PSITTACI

Chlam. psittaci infects a wide variety of animals. The most dangerous from the point of view of human infection are chlamydial infections in birds. Infected birds often, but not always, show signs of disease and this is known as *ornithosis*. When the birds belong to the psittacine family (e.g. budgerigars and parrots) the disease is known as *psittacosis*. The human disease is also called psittacosis—even if it has been acquired from non-psittacine birds: the majority of human cases are, in fact, acquired from pet budgerigars or parrots.

In Britain, psittacosis is a rare disease although the incidence has risen in recent years. Outbreaks of infection involving veterinary surgeons and workers in processing plants have been traced to infected flocks of ducks.

Psittacosis

Clinically: psittacosis most often takes the form of a *primary atypical pneumonia*: the patients have fever, cough and dyspnoea with extensive opacities in the lung fields on chest X-ray. Males are affected more often than females. The disease ranges in severity from a mild influenza-like illness to a severe disease with generalized toxaemic features. Psittacosis is sometimes fatal although the case fatality rate is low (probably less than 1%). Rarely, psittacosis may cause infective endocarditis, as well as myocarditis and pericarditis: renal involvement and disseminated intravascular coagulation are occasional complications.

Treatment: tetracycline.

Diagnosis

Serology

(i) *Complement fixation test*—for rising titre against the chlamydial common group antigen

(ii) *Immunofluorescence.*

20 Rickettsial diseases

Rickettsiae are not viruses—in fact they are like bacteria in their properties. Traditionally, like chlamydia, they are diagnosed in virus laboratories.

The most notorious rickettsial disease is typhus—an epidemic scourge in conditions of poverty, malnutrition (e.g. the German concentration camps of the Second World War) and of armies in the field. Typhus played a major part in the disintegration of Napoleon's army in the retreat from Moscow.

There are two genera within the family of rickettsiae:

1. Rickettsia
2. Coxiella.

The main difference between them is that coxiellae are resistant to drying.

RICKETTSIAE

Diseases due to organisms in this genus are world-wide in distribution but are not found in Britain. The main diseases are listed in Table 20.1.

Clinical features

Acute febrile illness with rash: the rash is usually maculopapular, occasionally vesicular. Rickettsial infections are generally severe diseases: haemorrhagic complications and lymphadenopathy are common.

Fatality rate: is often high in untreated cases (e.g. up to 20% with certain rickettsiae): with antibiotic treatment, the mortality is low.

Table 20.1 Rickettsial diseases

	Typhus group		Spotted fever group	Tsutsugamushi group
Disease	Typhus	Murine typhus	Rocky Mountain fever; other tick-borne fevers	Scrub typhus (tsutsugamushi fever)
Geographical distribution	World-wide	World-wide	World-wide	Far East
Causal organism	R. prowazeki	R. tyhi	R. rickettsii, R.conorii, R. sibirica, R. australis R. akari	R. tsutsugamushi
Vector	Louse	Flea	Ticks (mites with R. akari)	Mites
Reservoir	Man, flying squirrels (USA)	Rats	Ticks (mites with R. akari)	Mites
Weil-Felix reaction				
Proteus OX:19	+	+	+*†	—
Proteus OX:K	—	—	—	+
Proteus OX:2	—	—	+†	—

*Variable.
†no reaction with R. akari

Rickettsial pox: due to *R. akari* is a mite-borne milder rickettsial disease characterized by a vesicular rash: there is a papule at the site of the bite which progresses to an eschar. The rash with *R. australis*—a spotted fever found in Australia—also becomes vesicular.

Recurrent infection (Brill-Zinsser disease) is seen with classical typhus: recrudescences may be years after the primary illness and are usually mild.

Treatment: tetracycline or chloramphenicol.

Vectors: rickettsiae are transmitted to man via infected arthropods, e.g. ticks, lice and fleas. There is no human case-to-case transmission. Arthropods infect man by biting or by contamination of skin scratches with infected faeces (e.g. in typhus and murine typhus).

Reservoirs: usually the arthropod vectors, sometimes small animals, e.g. rodents (Table 20.1).

Proteus: rickettsiae share O antigens with certain *Proteus* species. Rickettsial disease can be diagnosed (although the test is not very reliable) by detecting raised antibody titres in agglutination tests with appropriate *Proteus* strains: known as the Weil-Felix reaction (Table 20.1).

Bacteriology

1. Large (relative to viruses) coccobacilli approximately 300 nm in diameter
2. Can be seen by light microscope with Giemsa or Macchiavello's stain, the organisms staining purplish and red respectively.
3. Contain both DNA and RNA (unlike viruses)
4. Replicate intracellularly but by binary fission: best isolated in guinea pigs, mice, or the yolk sac of chick embryos
5. Rapidly killed by drying
6. Sensitive to chloramphenicol and tetracycline.

Diagnosis

Serology

1. Tests: indirect micro-immunofluorescence, indirect haemagglutination, ELISA, latex agglutination

2. Weil-Felix reaction lacks specificity and antibodies appear late in infection.

Isolation: rarely attempted.

Control

A vaccine has been developed but is not generally available for typhus: it contains the attenuated E strain of *R. prowazeki*. Genetically-engineered protein vaccines are being developed against typhus and Rocky Mountain spotted fever. Control of vectors can cut short an epidemic.

Q FEVER

Coxiella burneti, the only member of the genus Coxiella and an important human pathogen, is distributed world-wide—including in Britain. It is common in domestic animals and causes Q or 'query' fever. A sporadic disease in Britain, it was first described as an outbreak of respiratory disease amongst meat workers in Queensland, Australia.

Clinical features

Signs and symptoms: are of a pyrexia of unknown origin (PUO): headache (a prominent symptom) with fever, generalized aches and anorexia; the pulse is slow and a proportion of cases have enlargement of the liver with abnormal liver function tests; more rarely there may be splenomegaly; Q fever is a generalized septicaemic infection.

Pneumonia: about half the patients have the signs and symptoms of primary atypical pneumonia with patchy consolidation of the lungs on chest X-ray.

Duration: about 2 weeks but the course is sometimes prolonged for 4 or more weeks especially in patients over 40 years old.

Prognosis: is good and complete recovery is usual.

Infective endocarditis: rarely Q fever may be followed by chronic infection with involvement of the heart valves and the formation of vegetations. The signs and symptoms are similar to those of bacterial infective endocarditis i.e. fever, finger clubbing, anaemia, heart murmurs and splenomegaly. Liver enlargement is common;

the disease is seen in patients in whom the heart valves are damaged by rheumatic heart disease or congenital malformation; Q fever endocarditis is a much more serious disease than Q fever.

Treatment

Q fever can be successfully treated with tetracycline or chloramphenicol.

Endocarditis: requires long-term treatment with tetracycline; this tends to suppress rather than eradicate the organism and careful follow-up is necessary; replacement of the diseased heart valves by valve prostheses has greatly improved the prognosis and long-term survival can now be achieved.

Epidemiology

Animal reservoirs: infection is endemic in domestic sheep and cattle; ticks can also be infected and may play a role in spreading *Cox. burneti* amongst animals, although generally this is via inhalation or ingestion of infected dust, straw, pasture etc.

Geographical distribution: the disease is world-wide.

Route of human infection: mainly by handling infected animals or by inhalation of contaminated dust; placentas of infected animals are heavily contaminated; infection may also be spread by drinking unpasteurized, contaminated milk from infected cows, although this seems to be an unusual route.

Occupational hazard: workers who handle animals have an increased risk of Q fever but, even in them, the disease is relatively rare.

Sex incidence: the majority of patients are male—probably reflecting the occupational hazard.

Seasonal incidence: Q fever is more common in spring and the early summer months.

Bacteriology

Cox. burneti is similar to the rickettsiae in its properties but differs in being resistant to drying; it can be cultivated in the yolk sac of the chick embryo and infects laboratory animals, e.g. guinea pigs.

Diagnosis

Serology

Complement fixation test: with two different preparations of *Cox. burneti* as antigens:

1. *Phase 1 antigen*: freshly isolated strains of *Cox. burneti* give no reaction with sera of acute cases but react well with sera from patients with long-standing chronic infection (i.e. endo-carditis).
2. *Phase 2 antigen*: strains of *Cox. burneti* after repeated passage in or adaptation to eggs, react well with sera of acute cases as well as sera from long-standing infections.

Acute Q fever

Serology: complement fixation test with phase 2 antigen.

Q fever endocarditis

Serology: complement fixation test with both phase 1 and phase 2 antigens: patients have high—usually very high—titres of antibodies to both antigens.

Isolation: by inoculation of guinea pigs with material from valvular vegetations and spleen: after an interval the guinea pig sera are tested for antibodies to *Cox. burneti* by complement fixation test.

Direct demonstration *of Cox. burneti* in smears on vegeta-tions on heart valves (taken at operation for valve replacement) and stained with Macchiavello's stain: *Cox. burneti* is detected as minute red coccobacilli.

21 Mycoplasma

There are three genera of mycoplasma:

1. Mycoplasma
2. Ureoplasma
3. Acholeplasma.

Mycoplasma can grow on inanimate bacteriological media. They are in fact bacteria which lack the peptidoglycan cell wall characteristic of bacteria.

The most important human pathogen in the group is *Mycoplasma pneumoniae*. Because it causes a disease long regarded as 'virus pneumonia', it is traditionally handled in virus laboratories.

MYCOPLASMA PNEUMONIAE

Clinical features

Respiratory infections

M. pneumoniae is primarily a respiratory pathogen. Although many, probably most, of the infections it causes are mild or even symptomless, it is an important cause of lower respiratory disease.

1. *Primary atypical pneumonia*: formerly known as 'virus pneumonia', with symptoms of fever, hacking non-productive cough and often a severe headache: marked weakness and tiredness are common. On X-ray there is patchy consolidation of the lungs. On average the disease lasts for about ten days but in a proportion of cases symptoms persist for considerably longer. Primary atypical pneumonia is also caused—but more rarely—by *Coxiella burneti* and *Chlamydia psittaci*.

2. *Other respiratory diseases*: M. *pneumoniae* also causes febrile bronchitis and tracheitis. Upper respiratory tract infection such as sinusitis, pharyngitis, coryza and otitis media (bullous myringitis) —and symptomless infection—are also common: most are not diagnosed in the laboratory.

Non-respiratory diseases

1. *Mucocutaneous eruptions*: M. *pneumoniae* also causes various types of rash—erythematous, maculopapular or vesicular. In a proportion of cases this is associated with conjunctival and mouth ulceration—the *Stevens-Johnson syndrome*.

2. *Neurological*: signs of CNS involvement are not uncommon in M. *pneumoniae* infection. These most often take the form of meningism, aseptic meningitis or meningo-encephalitis but cerebellar syndromes, transverse myelitis and nerve palsies have been reported.

3. *Haematological*: haemolytic anaemia sometimes complicates severe M. *pneumoniae* infection. This is probably due to the development of 'cold agglutinins'—a diagnostic feature of the disease (see below).

Epidemiology

M. *pneumoniae* infections are endemic in the community but approximately every four years there is an   extensive epidemic (doubtless reflecting waning herd immunity after the previous outbreak). The last epidemic in Britain was in the winter of 1986–87: the next epidemic is expected in the winter of 1990–91.

Season: M. *pneumoniae* is a winter pathogen.

Age: most patients are children or young adults: infection in the middle-aged or elderly is rare.

Diagnosis

Serology: three tests are used:

1. *Complement fixation test* for demonstration of rising titre or—more often—stationary high titres (i.e. 256 or over)
2. *Immunofluorescence* to demonstrate specific IgM
3. *Cold agglutinins*: patients commonly develop a haemagglutinin for human group O erythrocytes which acts at 4°C. This

interesting antibody seems to be produced as a result of antigenic sharing between *M. pneumoniae* and an antigen of human erythrocytes.

Treatment

Tetracycline; erythromycin in children.

OTHER MYCOPLASMA

Various mycoplasma species inhabit human hosts as commensals:

M. hominis—genital tract
M. orale—mouth
M. salivarius—mouth.

    M. orale and *M. salivarius* do not appear to be pathogenic. *M. hominis* can cause sepsis post-partum, post-abortion and in the neonate.

Ureoplasma

Sometimes known as T (or tiny) strain mycoplasmas. *Ureoplasma ureolyticum* is a commensal of the human genital tract. It is believed to cause a proportion of cases of non-gonococcal urethritis.

Acholeplasma

There are seven species within this genus: none are human pathogens.

RECOMMENDED READING

Collier L H Timbury M C (eds) 1990 Topley and Wilson's
principles of bacteriology, virology and immunity, 8th edn. Vol
4, Virology. Arnold, London

Grist, N R, Ho-Yen D O, Walker E, Williams G R 1988 Diseases
of infection. Oxford University Press.

Zuckerman A J, Banatuala J E, Pattison J R (eds) 1982 Principles
and practice of clinical virology. John Wiley & Sons, Chichester

Index

Page numbers in italics refer to Figures and tables.

Acholeplasma, 183, 185
Acupuncture, 128-9
Acute necrotizing encephalitis, 96
Acyclovir, 100, 103, 137-8
Adenoviruses, 53-6, 73
  clinical features, 53-4
  diagnosis, 55-6
  faecal, 53, 54
  oncogenic, 54
  persistent infection, 54
  respiratory syndromes, *54*
  virology, 54-5
Adsorption, 15
Aedes aegypti, 81
AIDS, 161-8
  antiviral drug, *137*
  clinical features, 162-4
  epidemiology, 166-7
  heterosexuals in sub-Saharan
    Africa, 166
  HIV-2 related, 164
  infections associated with, *163*
  Kaposi's sarcoma, *Plate 7*, 140
    163, 164
  opportunist infection treatment,
    168
  paediatric, 165
  risk factors, 166
  zidovudine therapy, 139
Alimentary
  papilloma, 151
  tract faecal adenoviruses, 54
Alphaherpesvirus, 98, 103
Alphavirus, 77
  virology, 82-3
Alzheimer's disease, 146

Amantadine, 140
Anti HBc, 132
Anti-P24 antibody, 162
Antibody, 9
  antiviral effects, 9
  capture tests, 31
  titre, 29
Antibody-dependent
  cell-mediated cytotoxicity, 9
  cellular cytolysis (ADCC), 11
Antigenic
  drift, 44
  shift, 43-4
  structure of influenza virus, 42-4
  variation, 43
Antiviral drugs, 12-13, 137-40
Arboviruses, 77
  classification, *78*
  diagnosis, 84
  encephalitis, 77, 78-9
  fever with haemorrhage, 77, 79-84
  vaccines, 84
  virology, 82-4
Arenavirus, 92-4
Argentinian haemorrhagic fever, 93-4
Arthropod-borne infections, 77-84
  disease, 77, *78*
  hosts, 77
  rickettsial, *178*, 179, 180
  tick-borne encephalitis, 84
  vectors, 7, 77
Aseptic meningitis, 57, 58
  enteroviral, 63
Assembly, 16
  of DNA genomes and proteins, 21
  parainfluenza virus, 25
  poliovirus, 22
  retrovirus, 27
Astrovirus, 72-3

B19 virus, 120-2
B-lymphocytes, 9
Baltimore classification, 19
Betaherpesvirus, 106
BK virus, 141, 142, 143
Bolivian haemorrhagic fever, 93-4
Bone marrow transplant, 54, 105
Bornholm disease, 64
Bovine
    papilloma virus type, 4 151
    spongiform encephalopathy (BSE),
        145
Bracken, 151
Brill-Zinsser disease, 179
Bronchiolitis
    parainfluenza viruses, 48
    respiratory syncytial virus, 49-50
Bunyavirus, 77, 82, 94
    virology, 83-4
Burkitt's lymphoma, 107, 108-9
Butcher's warts, 150

Calcivirus, 69, 70, 73-4
California encephalitis, 78, 79
Cancer
    and AIDS, 164
    cervical, 151-2
    Epstein-Barr virus, 107, 108-9
    hepatitis B, 130
    natural, 155
    papilloma viruses, 150-1
    retrovirus oncogenes, 156-7
    retroviruses, 155, 158-9
    skin, 152
    viral cause, 168
    see also Oncogenicity
Cannibalism, 147
Capsid, 2
Capsomeres, 2
Carcinoma-in-situ see Cervical
    intraepithelial neoplasia (CIN)
Cardiac abnormalities, 117
Cataract, 116, 117
CD4 receptors, 159
Cell
    death, 3
    effects of viruses, 3-4
    mediated immune response to
        virus, 10
    transformation, 3
Cellular immunity, 9, 10-11
Central nervous system (CNS)
    Mycoplasma pneumoniae infection,
        185
    viral disease, 57-60

Cervical
    cancer, 151-2
    intraepithelial neoplasia (CIN), 151
Chemotherapy, antiviral, 12-13
Chick embryo
    cultivation, 3
    growth in amniotic cavity, 42
    influenza diagnosis, 45
    in virus diagnosis, 36
Chickenpox, 100, 101
Chikungunya, 78, 81
Childhood fevers, 111-22
Chlamydia
    antibiotic sensitivity, 170
    bacteriology, 170
Chlamydia pneumoniae, 169, 173-4
Chlamydia psittaci, 169, 174-5, 183
Chlamydia trachomatis, 169, 170-3
    diagnosis, 173
    lymphogranuloma venereum, 172
    non-specific genital infection, 170-1
    ocular infection, 171-2
    pneumonia, 172
Chlamydial disease, 169-75
Chloramphenicol, 179, 181
Chloroform, 6
Chronic neurological virus diseases,
        141-7
    progressive multifocal
        leucoencephalopathy, 141-3
    subacute sclerosing
        panencephalitis, 141
    unconventional agents, 143-7
Classification, 4, 5, 6
    arboviruses, 78
    Baltimore, 19
    gastroenteritis viruses, 69, 70
Coe virus see Coxsackievirus
Cold
    agglutinins, 184
    effects, 5
Cold sores, 98, 100
    acyclovir therapy, 138
Common cold, 56
Complement fixation test, 32
    influenza diagnosis, 44
Condylomata acuminata, 149, 151
Congo/Crimean haemorrhagic fever,
        82
Conjunctival defence mechanism, 8
Conjunctivitis, 53, 96
Contagious pustular dermatitis, 124
Continuous cell lines, 34
Coronavirus, 56
Coxiella burneti, 180, 181-2, 183
Coxiellae, 177, 180-2

Coxsackievirus, 56, 61
  Danish outbreak (1930), 64
  diagnosis, 66
  herpangina, 63
  myocarditis, 64
  pericarditis, 64
  rash, 63
Cranial zoster, 102
Creutzfeldt-Jakob disease, 59, 143,
  145-6
Cultivation of viruses, 2-3
Cytomegalic inclusion disease, 104-5
Cytomegalovirus, 95, 103-6
  antiviral drug, 137
  congenital, 104-5
  ganciclovir therapy, 139
  latency, 104
  owl's eye inclusion, 104, 106
  postnatal, 105-6
  treatment, 106
  virology, 106
Cytopathic effect (CPE), 35
Cytotoxic lymphocytes see T_c cells

Defence mechanism
  non-specific, 7, 8
  specific-immunological, 9-11
Delayed type hypersensitivity cells see
  T_d cells
Delta agent see Hepatitis D
Dementia, AIDS related, 164
Dengue, 78, 81
  haemorrhagic shock syndrome, 81
  vaccine, 84
Diarrhoea, 69
  virus, 75
Direct demonstration
  influenza diagnosis, 45
  parainfluenza viruses, 49
  respiratory syncytial virus, 51
  of virus, 29, 37
Diseases, 4-6, 7
Disinfectants, viral, 7
Dog vaccines, 90
Double-stranded
  DNA virus, 19-20
  RNA virus replication, 25-6
Drug abuse, 128, 132, 134, 135
  AIDS risk, 166, 167
  HTLV-2, 161
Drying effects, 5

Ebola virus, 85, 90-2
Echovirus, 56, 61

Electron microscopy
  astrovirus diagnosis, 73
  in direct demonstration of virus,
    37
  Norwalk virus diagnosis, 74
  rotavirus diagnosis, 72
Encephalitis, 57, 58, 77, 78-9
  acyclovir therapy, 138
  measles complication, 114
  rabies, 85
Endocarditis, 181, 182
Enteroviruses, 56, 61-7
  clinical features, 62
  diagnosis, 65-7
  diseases, 62
  epidemiology, 64-5
  groups, 61
  neurological syndromes, 62-3
  non-neurological syndromes, 63-4
  properties, 61
  vaccination, 67
  virology, 65
Entry, 15
  to body, 7
Envelope, 2
Enzyme-linked immunoabsorbent
  assay (ELISA), 30-1
Epidemic myalgia see Bornholm
  disease
Epidermodysplasia verruciformis,
  149-50, 151
  squamous cell carcinoma, 152
Epstein-Barr virus, 95, 106-7, 108-9
  antibody, 108
  virology, 109
Equine encephalitis, 78, 79
  vaccine, 84
Erythema infectiosum, 120-2
  clinical features, 121
  diagnosis, 122
  epidemiology, 121-2
  virology, 122
Erythromycin, 170, 171, 185
Ether, 6
Exanthema subitum, 110

Factor VIII
  hepatatis C contamination, 134
  HIV contamination, 167
Faecal viruses, 37
Feline leukaemia virus, 156
Fetus
  B19 infection, 121
  cytomegalovirus infection, 104
  varicella infection, 101

Fever with haemorrhage, arbovirus, 77, 79-84
Fibrosarcoma, 158
Fifth disease *see* Erythema infectiosum
Flavivirus, 77
  virology, 83
Foscarnet, 106

Gammaherpesvirus, 109
Ganciclovir, 106, 139
Gastroenteritis, 37, 69-75
  classification of viruses, 69, *70*
  clinical features, 69-70
  epidemiology, 70-1
  treatment, 71
  viruses, 71-4
Generalized herpes infection, 97
Genes, retrovirus, 156-7, 158
Genital herpes, 95, 97, 100
  acyclovir therapy, 138
Genital warts, *Plate 6*, 149, 150
Genome, 1, 16, *17*, 18-19
  fragmented, 25
Gingivo-stomatitis, 96
Glandular fever *see* Infectious mononucleosis
Gluteraldehyde, 7
Growth cycle of virus, 15-16
Guillain-Barré syndrome, 45-6

Haemadsorption, 4, 35, *36*
  influenza diagnosis, 45
Haemagglutination
  by influenza viruses, 42
  erythrocytes, 42
  in influenza diagnosis, 45
  parainfluenza viruses, 49
  test, 35, *36*
Haemagglutination-inhibition
  and influenza virus typing, 45
  strain-specific, 42
  test, 33
Haemagglutinin, 41, 42
  antigenic change, 43
  antigenic drift, 44
  replacement in antigenic shift, 43
  strain-specific, 43
Haemophiliacs, 132, 134
  HIV infection in children, 165
  HIV-1 infection, 167
Haemophilus influenzae, 40
Haemorrhagic
  conjunctivitis, 64

fever with renal syndrome (HFRS), 94
Hairy leukoplakia of tongue, 163
Hantaan virus, 94
Hantavirus, 77, 83
HBsAg, 132, 133
Heat effects, 5
Helper lymphocyte *see* T$_h$ cells
Hepatitis, 105
  anicteric, 126
  chronic, 126, 129-30
  chronic active, 134
  post-transfusion, 133-4
  water-borne, 136
Hepatitis A, 126, 126-8
Hepatitis B, 126, 128-33
  animal counterparts, 129
  antigenic structure, 131-2
  cancer, 130
  carriers, 129
  core antigen antibody, 132
  diagnosis, 132-3
  epidemiology, 128-9
  and hepatitis D, 135
  non-parenteral spread, 129
  sequelae, 129-30
  subtype distribution of antigens, 132
  surface antigen antibody, 132
  vaccine, 133
  virology, 130
  virus, *131*
  virus replication, 21
Hepatitis C, 126, 133-5
Hepatitis D, 135
Hepatitis E, 135-6
  antigen clearance by interferon, 140
Hepatitis, viral, 125-36
  clinical features, 125-6
  complications, 126
Hepatocellular carcinoma, 130, 134
Herpangina, 63
Herpes
  hepatitis, 97
  neonatal infection, 97
Herpes simplex virus, 95-100
  antiviral drug, 137, 138
  clinical features, 96-8
  diagnosis, 100
  epidemiology, 98
  latency, 97
  neutralizing antibody, 97
  primary infections, *Plate 3*, 96-7
  reactivation, 97, 98
  replication, 19

Herpes simplex virus (contd)
  treatment, 100
  virology, 98-9
Herpes zoster, 100
Herpesvirus diseases, 95-110
Herpetic whitlow, 96
Homosexuals, 128, 132
  AIDS risk, 166
  Kaposi's sarcoma, 164
Horses, arbovirus encephalitis, 79
Host response to infection, 7-11
HTLV-1, 159, 160-1
  associated myelopathy, 160
HTLV-2, 161
Human
  cancer viral cause, 168
  diploid cell vaccine (HDCV), 89, 90
  herpes virus 6, 95, 109-10
  papillomavirus virus, 151, 152
  parvovirus B19, 120-2
  T-cell lymphotropic retrovirus, 159
Human immunodeficiency virus
  (HIV), 161-8
  clinical features, 162-4
  diagnosis, 167
  epidemiology, 166-7
  mother to baby transmission, 165
  treatment, 168
  virology, 167
Human immunodeficiency virus
  (HIV-1), 159
  haemophiliac infection, 167
Human immunodeficiency virus
  (HIV-2), 159
  infection, 164
Human retroviruses, 159-68
  clinical features, 160, 162-4
  diagnosis, 161
  epidemiology, 160-1
  virology, 161
Hydrops fetalis, 121
Hypochlorite solution, 7

Idoxuridine, 100, 138
IgA, 9
IgG, 9, 11
  ELISA test, 31
IgM, 9
  detection, 29
  ELISA test, 30, 31
IgM antibody
  capture tests, 31
  and rubella syndrome, 117
Immunization
  hepatitis A, 128

hepatitis B, 133
  prophylactic, 88-9
Immunofluorescence, 36, 37
  influenza diagnosis, 45
  tests, 32
Immunoglobulin, 9
  normal, 116
Immunological responses
  cellular, 9, 10-11
  humoral, 8, 9
Immunosuppression, cytomegalovirus
  infection, 105
Immunosuppressive therapy, 98, 100
  MMR vaccination, 120
Inclusion
  blennorrhoea, 171
  bodies, 37
  conjunctivitis, 171
Infant mortality, 69
Infection
  host response, 7-11
  latent, 3-4
Infectious mononucleosis, 105, 107-9
Infectivity, 18-19
Influenza, 39-46
  antiviral drug, 137
  clinical features, 39
  complications, 39-40
  diagnosis, 44-5
  epidemics, 40, 41
  epidemiology, 40-1
  mutant strain, 44
  pandemics, 39, 41, 43-4
  strains, 44
  vaccines, 45-6
  virology, 41-2
  virus antigenic structure, 42-4
  virus types, 40
Influenza A, amantadine therapy, 140
Ingestion, 7
Inhalation, 7
Inoculation, 7
Interferon, 11-13, 140
  antiviral activity, 12
  antiviral chemotherapy, 12-13
  defence mechanism, 8
Interleukin-1 (IL-1), 10
Invasiveness, 7
Isolation
  adenovirus diagnosis, 55-6
  enteroviruses, 65-6
  influenza diagnosis, 44
  parainfluenza viruses, 49
  respiratory syncytial virus, 51
  rhinoviruses, 53
  of virus, 29

Japanese B encephalitis, 78
vaccine, 84
Jaundice, 125, 126
JC virus, 141, 142
Jenner E, 123
Junin virus, 92, 93, 94

Kaposi's sarcoma, 163, 164
with AIDS, *Plate 7*
interferon therapy, 140
Kaposi's varicelliform eruption, 96
Keratitis, 96, 98, 100
Kerato-conjunctivitis, epidemic, 54
Killer (K) cells, 11
Kuru, *59*, *143*, 146-7
Kyasanur Forest fever, 81

Laboratory animal
cultivation, 3
inoculation, 37
Laboratory diagnosis, 29-37
direct demonstration, 37
serology, 29-33
virus isolation, 33-7
Laryngeal papilloma, 149, 150
Lassa fever
ribavirin therapy, 139
virus, 92, 93, 94
Latent infection, 3-4
Leukaemia, 155
virus, 158-9
Liver necrosis, massive, 126
Louping ill, 79
Lymphocytic choriomeningitis, 92, 94
Lymphogranuloma venereum, 172
Lyssavirus, 87

Machupo virus, 92, 93
Macrophages, activated, 11
Major histocompatibility antigens
(MHC), Class II, 10
Malaria and EB virus, 108, 109
Malignant lymphoma, 108
Marburg virus, 85, 90-2
Measles, 113-16
clinical features, 113-14
diagnosis, 115
epidemiology, 114-15
neurological complications, 114
respiratory infection, 113-14
vaccination, 111, 115, 116, 119-20
virology, 115

Meningitis *see* Aseptic meningitis
Metabolic activity, 1
Microcephaly, 104
MMR vaccine *see* Vaccination,
measles, mumps and rubella
(MMR)
Molluscum contagiosum, 123
Monkey kidney tissue culture, 42
inoculation in influenza diagnosis,
44-5
parainfluenza viruses, 49
Monkeypox, 124
Mononucleosis, 107
with cervical lymphadenopathy, 110
Motor neurone disease, 146
Multiple sclerosis, 146
Mumps, 111-13
clinical features, 111-12
diagnosis, 112-13
epidemiology, 112
meningitis, 111
vaccination, 111, 119-20
Murray Valley encephalitis, 78
Mycoplasma, 183-5
T strain, 185
Mycoplasma hominis, 185
Mycoplasma orale, 185
Mycoplasma pneumoniae, 183-5
CNS involvement, 184
haemolytic anaemia, 184
mucocutaneous eruptions, 184
non-respiratory diseases, 184
respiratory diseases, 183-4
Mycoplasma salivarius, 185
Myocarditis, 64

Nairovirus, 77, 83
Nasopharyngeal carcinoma, 107, 109
Natural killer (NK) cells, 11
Negri bodies, 86, 88
Neonatal
herpes infection, 97
ophthalmia, 171
Nerve deafness, 117
Neuralgia, 102
Neuraminidase, 41, 42
immunity to reinfection, 43
replacement in antigenic shift,
43
Neurological disease, 57-60
acute viral, 57, *58*, 60
chronic viral, *59*, 60
enteroviral, 62-3
syndromes, 57, *59*

Neutralization, 9
  tests, 33
Non-structured viruses (SRVs), 69,
  71, 74
Normal immunoglobulin, 116
Norwalk virus, 69, 70, 71, 74
Nucleic acid, 2, 16
Nucleocapsid, 42
Nucleoprotein, 42

Oinyon-nyong, 81
Oncogenes, 156-7
  activation, 157
Oncogenicity, 168
  adenovirus, 54
  see also Cancer
Orf, 124
Ornithosis, 174
Oropouche, 82
Orthomyxoviruses, 41
Owl's eye inclusion, 104, 106
Oxidizing agents, 6

P24, 162
Papilloma virus
  cervical cancer, 151-2
  human cancer, 151
  malignant change, 150-1
  type, 150
  type 18 DNA, 151
Parainfluenza virus, 48-9
  assembly, 25
  clinical features, 48
  diagnosis, 49
  replication, 24-5
  transcription, 25
  virology, 48-9
  virus protein synthesis, 25
  virus RNA synthesis, 25
Paralysis, 57, 58
  enteroviral, 63
Paramyxoviruses, 48
Paravaccinia, 124
Parvovirus replication, 21
Pasteur L, 88
Paul-Bunnell test, 107-8, 109
Pericarditis, 64
Phagocytosis, 8
Pharyngitis, 53
Phenols, 7
Phlebovirus, 77, 83
Picornavirus, 52, 65
Plantar warts, 149, 150

Pleurodynia see Bornholm disease
Pneumonia
  antiviral drug, 137
  Chlamydia pneumoniae, 174
  Chlamydia trachomatis, 172
  cytomegalovirus, 105
  giant cell, 114
  parainfluenza viruses, 48
  primary atypical, 183
  primary influenzal, 39-40
  psittacosis, 174
  respiratory syncytial virus, 49-50
  secondary bacterial, 40
Pneumovirus, 51
Poliomyelitis
  enteroviral, 63
  paralysis, Plate 1
Poliovirus
  assembly, 24
  replication, 22-4
  translation, 22
  virus RNA synthesis, 23-4
Polymerase chain reaction (PCR)
  technique, 37
Polymorphonuclear leucocytes, 11
Polyoma replication, 19
Post-infectious encephalomyelitis, 57,
  58, 60
Poxvirus diseases, 123-4
Pregnancy
  cytomegalovirus infection, 103, 104
  hepatitis E, 136
  MMR vaccination, 120
  rubella, 116, 117, 118, 119
  varicella infection, 101
  viruria with JC and BK viruses, 143
Primary
  site of influenza virus
    multiplication, 39
  tissue cultures, 34
Prions, 145
Probes, 37
Progressive multifocal
  leucoencephalopathy, 59, 141-3
B-Propiolactone, 7
Protein coat, 1
Proteus, 179
Pseudocowpox, 124
Psittacosis, 174-5
Purtillo's syndrome, 108

Q fever, 180-2
  bacteriology, 181
  clinical features, 180-1

Q fever (*contd*)
  diagnosis, 182
  endocarditis, 181, 182
  epidemiology, 181

Rabies, 57, 85-90
  clinical features, 85-6
  diagnosis, 88
  dumb, 85-6
  epidemiology, 86-7
  furious, 85
  hydrophobic spasm, *Plate 2*
  vaccination, 88-90
  virology, 87-8
Radial immune haemolysis, 33
Radio-immune assay (RIA), 31
Ramsay Hunt syndrome, 102
Receptors of influenza virus, 42
Reducing agents, 6
Reiter's syndrome, 170
Release, 16
Renal dialysis, 129
Renal transplant, 105
  squamous cell carcinoma risk, 152
  warts, 152
Reovirus replication, 25-6
Replication biochemistry, 19-27
Respiratory diseases, 183-4
Respiratory syncytial virus, 49-51
  antiviral drug, *137*
  clinical features, 49-50
  diagnosis, 51
  epidemiology, 50-1
  immunopathology, 50
  ribavirin therapy, 140
  virology, 51
Respiratory tract defence mechanism,
  8
Respiratory tract infections, 47-56
  adenovirus, 53-6
  common cold, 56
  parainfluenza, 48-9
  respiratory syncytial virus, 49-51
  rhinovirus, 51-3
  viruses, *47*
  see also Influenza
Retrovirus, 155-68
  animal tumour-producing, *159*
  assembly, 27
  endogenous, 158
  epidemiology, 157
  genome, 26, 156, 158
  morphology, 155
  natural cancer, 155

  oncogenes, 156-7
  particles, 155
  replication, 26-7
  transmission, 157-8
  tumours produced by, 158-9
  virus protein synthesis, 26
  see also Human retroviruses
Reye's syndrome, 40
Rhabdovirus, 87
Rhinovirus, 51-3
  clinical features, 51-2
  diagnosis, 53
  epidemiology, 52
  virology, 52-3
Ribavirin, 139-40
Rickettsiae, 177-80
  bacteriology, 179
  diagnosis, 179-80
  vaccination, 180
Rickettsial diseases, 177-82
  Q fever, 180-2
  recurrent infection, 179
  spotted fever, *178*, 179, 180
  typhus, 177, *178*, 179, 180
  vectors, 179, 180
Rickettsial pox, 179
Rift Valley fever, 82
mRNA, 1
  probes in detection, 37
  virus, 15, 16
RNA virus, 41
  parainfluenza, 48
  replication, 22-7
Rociovirus, 78
Rocky Mountain Spotted fever, *178*,
  180
Roseola infantum *see* Exanthema
  subitum
Ross River virus, 82
Rotavirus, 71-2
Rous sarcoma virus replication, 26-7
Rubella, 116-19
  congenital infection, *Plate 5*, 116-17
  diagnosis, 118-19
  epidemiology, 117-18
  immunity, 33, 117
  syndrome, 117
  vaccination, 111, 119-20
  virology, 118

S soluble antigen, 42-3
Sabin live attenuated virus vaccine, 67
St Louis encephalitis, 78, 79
Salk inactivated virus vaccine, 67

Sarcoma, 155
  virus, 158
Sclerosing panencephalitis, subacute, 59
Scrapie, *143*, 144-5
Semi-continuous cell strains, 34
Semple vaccine, 89
Serological tests,
  immunofluorescence, 37
Serology, 29-33
  adenovirus diagnosis, 55-6
  arbovirus diagnosis, 84
  enteroviruses, 66-7
  influenza diagnosis, 44
  parainfluenza viruses, 49
  respiratory syncytial virus, 51
  rhinoviruses, 53
  rotavirus diagnosis, 72
  tests, 30-3
  yellow fever diagnosis, 80
Severe generalized cytomegalovirus
  infection, 104-5
Shingles, 100, 101
Shope papilloma, 151
Single-stranded
  negative sense RNA virus, 24-5
  positive sense RNA virus, 22-4
Size of viruses, 1
Skin
  cancer, 152
  defence mechanism, 8
Slapped cheek disease *see* Erythema
  infectiosum
Slim disease, 164
Slow virus diseases, 141
Small round structured virus
  (SRSVs), 69, 74
Smallpox, 123
Squamous
  cell carcinoma, 150, 152
  epithelioma, 149
Staphylococcus aureus, 40
Stevens-Johnson syndrome, 184
Structure of viruses, 1-2
Subacute sclerosing panencephalitis,
  114, 117, *141*
Suckling mouse brain vaccine, 90
Sulphonamides, 172
Suppressor lymphocytes *see* T$_S$ cells
Symmetry of virus particles, 2
Synthesis of virus components, 16

T4 helper lymphocytes, HIV
  cytopathic effect, 161

T4 lymphocyte, 159
  in AIDS, 162, 164
T-cell leukaemia/lymphoma, 160
T-helper cells, 9, 10-11
Taiwan acute respiratory agent
  (TWAR) *see* Chlamydia
  pneumoniae
Tanapox, 124
Tattooing, 128-9
T$_c$ cells, 10-11
T$_d$ cells, 11
Temperature effects, 5
Tetracycline, 170, 171, 172, 175,
  179, 181
  Mycoplasma penumoniae treatment,
  185
T$_h$ cells, 10
Tick-borne encephalitis vaccine, 84
Tissue culture, 3, 34-6
  virus growth, 35-6
Trachoma, *Plate 8*, 171-2
Track runners, 129
Transcription, 15-16, *18*
  double-stranded DNA virus, 19
  parainfluenza virus, 25
Translation, poliovirus, 22
Transmissible mink encephalopathy,
  145
Tropical spastic paraparesis, *159*, 160
T$_s$ cells, 10
Tsutsugamushi fever, *178*
Typhus, 177, *178*, 179
  vaccination, 180

Ultra-violet irradiation, 6
Uncoating, 15
Ureoplasma, 183, 185
Urethritis, 185
Urinary tract defence mechanism, 8
Uukuvirus, 77, 83

Vaccination
  arboviruses, 84
  enteroviruses, 67
  hepatitis B, 133
  influenza, 45-6
  Junin virus, 94
  measles, mumps and rubella
  (MMR), 111, 112, 116, 119-20
  pre-exposure, 90
  rabies, 8-90
  rickettsiae, 180
  typhus, 180

Vaccinia, 124
  replication, 19
Varicella, 100-2
  epidemiology, 101-2
  vidarabine therapy, 139
Varicella-zoster
  antiviral drug, 137, 138
  virus, 95, 100-3
Vectors *see* Arthropod-borne
  infections
Vibrio cholerae, 42
Vidarabine, 139
Viraemia, 63
Virion, 2, 19
Virus
  antibody detection, 29
  genome probes in detection, 37
  haemagglutinin, 42
  isolation, 33-7
  mRNA, 15, 16
  pneumonia *see* Pneumonia, primary
    atypical
  vaccines, 45-6
Virus DNA
  radioactive, 37
  synthesis, 19-20
  warts diagnosis, 153
Virus protein synthesis, 16, 20-1
  parainfluenza virus, 25
  retrovirus, 26
Virus RNA synthesis
  parainfluenza virus, 25
  poliovirus, 22

Virus-specific messenger, 1
Vomiting, 69, 70, 73, 74
Vulvar warts, malignant change, 151

Warts, 149-53
  cervical, 151
  clinical features, 149-50
  diagnosis, 153
  epidemiology, 150
  genital, *Plate 6*, 149, 150
  papillomavirus type, *150*
  tumour forming potential, 149, 150
  virology, 152-3
Weil-Felix reaction, *178*, 179
Winter vomiting disease, 70, 73
World Health Organization, 123

Yellow fever, 78, 80
  vaccine, 84

Zidovudine, 139, 168
Zoonoses, 85
Zoster, 102-3
  acyclovir prophylaxis, 138
  amantadine therapy, 140
  thoracic rash, *Plate 4*
  vidarabine therapy, 139